THE ANIMAL AROMATICS
WORKBOOK

Giving animals the choice to select their own natural medicines

Caroline Ingraham

with nutrition by Nick Thompson BSc (Hons), BVM&S, VetMFHom, MRCVS

This book may not be reproduced in whole or in part by any means without the expressed permission of the author. The author has asserted her right under the Copyright Design and Patent Act 1988 (and under any comparable provision of any comparable law in any jurisdiction whatsoever) to be identified as the author of this work.
So far as may legally effectively be provided no liability of an kind or nature whatsoever, whether in negligence, under stature, or otherwise, is accepted by the author or the publisher for the accuracy or safety of the information or advice contained in, or in any way relating to the content of this material.

All rights reserved. No part of this publication may be reproduced, stored in a retrieval system, or transmitted in any form or by any means, electronic, mechanical, photocopying, recording, or otherwise, without the prior permission of the copyright holder.

ISBN: 0-9524827-11
ISBN: 978-0-9524827-1-0

Published by Caroline Ingraham
www.ingraham.co.uk

Copyright © 2006 Caroline Ingraham
All rights reserved

This book is dedicated to animals that have died for mankind and to my supportive children Thomas and Madeleine

SECOND EDITION

Book & cover design by Giles Morgans. www.pixelshifters.com
Back cover photo www.worldwidefeatures.com. Photographed at the WHF Kent.
Printed in England by Orphans Press, Hereford Road, Leominster, Herefordshire HR6 8JT.

The information in this book comes from practical experience and clinical research. It should not be substituted for veterinary advice. The author cannot be held responsible for the use of the oils or plant extracts and their application.

Useful information for products used in this book, education and information

Please contact
The Ingraham Institute, 9, Booth Gardens, Hay-on-Wye, Herefordshire HR3 5BH
Tel. 01497 822775 or 0845 257 0840
Email: caroline@ingraham.co.uk
www.ingraham.co.uk

foreword

Caroline Ingraham, as the longest practicing Animal Aromatics practitioner in the UK, is in an ideal position to write this valuable book. Not only does she draw from her twenty year experience, she brings us research in her field to back up her work.

I found this book fascinating. In it she deals with conditions that are very difficult to treat satisfactorily and fully using conventional medicine. Used carefully, in consultation with an Animal Aromatics practitioner and veterinary surgeon, this book could help countless animals. I applaud her hard work and generosity in codifying the responsible use of Animal Aromatics in the veterinary sphere.

Nick Thompson BSc.(Hons), BVM&S, VetMFHom, MRCVS.

acknowledgments

I feel I that I should mention Cindy Engel first for her inspirational book ' Wild Health', that took me deeper into the journey of Animal Aromatics. Her scientific evidence supported my observational research with captive animals. I learnt a lot - thank you Cindy.

I would like to say a heart-felt thank you to Rhiannon Harris who painstakingly went through hours of essential oil science edits to make sure that the information given was as scientifically correct as possible, searching for references to support my many claims. The book owes much to her behind the scenes work and support.

I would also like to thank Giles Morgans for all the thought and care he put into the book design and its cover; and for putting up with my many edits - thank you Giles. My thanks also extend to Nick Thompson whom from the day I met him at an Holistic Veterinary Medicine conference in 1999 has had an open mind to Animal Aromatics, respecting and embracing its ethos; it is an honour to have him write on nutrition in this book. Sam Davis, too, has made a valuable contribution with her work on cats in a rescue cattery. Her work will clear up many misconceptions on essential oils being offered to cats - thank you Sam.

There is also my eighteen year old son Thomas to thank who has helped me put thoughts into words in certain parts of the book. His interest in animals was apparent from a very early age and he now intends to incorporate my work mingled with his own scientific studies, at University College London. I would also like to thank his little sister and my daughter Maddie who at the age of thirteen coped with the household chores without complaint, while I wrote this book.

Janet Mortimer and veterinary nurse Jenny Ward, both Animal Aromatic students, have also helped greatly with suggestions and structure of the book. Orphans Press should also be mentioned here for their personal support and help with self - publishing; and last but not least my many students and animals who have contributed their experiences in order to help others, in the same way as they have been helped by using the remedies mentioned in this book.

chapters

Acknowledgments	**4**
The aim of this book	**6**
Introduction	**7**
Aromatics and self selection	**10**
Pathways into the body	20
A step by step guide	**30**
Organ systems of the body	**50**
Base Materials	**61**
Minerals, algae & plant extracts	**66**
Essential oil profiles	**86**
First Aid	**152**
Common disorders	**155**
Working with different species	**158**
Equine	159
Canine	177
Feline	192
Rodents & rabbits	207
Avian	211
Farm animals	214
Exotics	219
Nutrition	**223**

the aim of this book

The purpose of this book is to give back to people the responsibility of helping their animals. Many of us have become removed from the privilege of understanding and knowing how to help ourselves, our children and our animals for minor medical problems as well as chronic disease. When we allow others to think and do for us, we begin to lose the innate knowledge that we hold within ourselves, and when this is lost we are more likely to make mistakes and have accidents.

At one time the use and understanding of essential oils, plants and their medicinal properties were common knowledge in the home and they were the medicines found in veterinary surgeons and doctors brief cases, (reference to their use can be found in Black's Veterinary Dictionary, published in 1928).
We are beginning to face a mounting toll of complications caused by over use of aggressively synthesised chemical medicines. We need to make a conscious effort to retain or regain what has always been our universal right and to take some responsibility for the health of ourselves, our children, and our animals. We need to reconsider the importance of natural medicine, combining, wisdom from the past and scientific knowledge from the present.

using this book

Reference charts and guides to specific essential oils and remedies for common ailments, provide suggestions of the way to use aromatics to look after the health of our animals. The book also provides a deeper understanding of how and why essential oils and remedies may work for particular conditions. The formulations and suggestions are not a substitute for veterinary advice and if in any doubt, readers should always consult a veterinary surgeon before using the plant extracts. It is important to understand and check the remedy that is being offered against the information in this book before offering it to the animal; as well as consulting the methods of selection and administration. Never apply a remedy to an animal without offering it first. If an animal shows any signs of rejecting it, do not apply. Essential oils and plant extracts are listed according to their common names, as readers may be unfamiliar with their Latin botanical name. They also appear in the text according to their common name.

introduction

The innate ability to self-select correct foods and medicines is vital for the survival of mammals in the wild. In field trips, scientists in search of raw materials for new pharmaceutical drugs are known to follow and closely observe how primates make their selection of medicinal plants within their natural environment. When the primates are seen to significantly alter their normal behaviour, stop eating and start to consume different herbs, the researchers know this is a sign to send these plants to the lab for analysis, as it is likely they will contain components that are possible new cures for humankind. Nearly 40% of our pharmaceuticals contain constituents originally found in the plant kingdom.

Cindy Engel[1] in her ground breaking book, *Wild Health* provides an excellent example of a primate self selecting a medicinal plant that was subsequently examined in the laboratory. 'A chimp that was clearly unwell, her urine was dark and discoloured, her stools loose and her back was quite obviously stiff, sought out a shrub (*Vernonia amygdalina*), which is commonly known as bitter-leaf and is so poisonous that locally it is called goat killer, but is also used medicinally to treat diseases such as malarial fever and amoebic dysentery. The extreme bitter taste of the aromatic fruit is normally a warning sign to stay away, but not for this sick chimp; she chewed and sucked on the inner pith for about 20 minutes. The sick mother, after ingesting her remedy took long naps for the remainder of the day and by the next day she was well on the mend. When the pith was analysed it was found to contain steroid glucosides, as well as four known sesquiterpene lactones capable of killing parasites, that could have produced the symptoms she was displaying'.

In 1984 I began my training in the use of essential oils. However, it was not from these studies that I gained my wealth of knowledge, it was from the animals themselves. I noticed that when an animal had been separated from a companion, or taken from its mother too early, it would select neroli, and animals from rescue homes would choose rose or linden blossom, and so the pattern evolved. Horses with respiratory disorders caused by allergies would select German chamomile or great mugwort. If the allergic reaction was severe, the animal would first select great mugwort, then as the condition began to clear, German chamomile would be chosen. Not only did I find that their selection had a definite pattern, but so did their application. Most oils offered for internal problems were taken by mouth, whereas oils for emotional problems were usually inhaled. The remedies that the animal selected taught me a a lot about its condition; if the problem was due to a bacterial infection, the animal would select antibacterial oils and so on.

After writing my first book, I had a wealth of knowledge on essential oils and horses but something was missing from my remedy kit for most carnivores. This lead me to research which of the remedies animals normally selected in the wild and how they themselves administered them. With this I could further understand domestic animal's needs and why they were selecting such plant extracts. For example: In the wild, dogs will generally drink from puddles and murky ponds where algae grows; which is not too different from the domestic dog that will usually choose rain or pond water over tap water. I have since discovered that dogs especially with afflictions such as skin allergies and arthritis will select spirulina (algae), which, literally in many cases, turns them around back to health very quickly; this is now offered to dogs almost as a matter of routine by those that work with the principles of Animal Aromatics.

I then began to observe how cats behave and liken that to the way they select their remedies; in the wild they roll on the plant which crushes it and releases its fragrance, which is then inhaled. Occasionally they will take plants by mouth. This is not too dissimilar to their selection and behaviour with aromatic extracts offered to them. It is the dried plants that they roll in, with a small selection of remedies that they may take by mouth, however, essential oils are usually only inhaled. Unlike mammals that generally eat plants, fruits and vegetables as part of their diet, cats will only eat plants for medicinal purposes.

Following the remarkable recovery of my dog that was bitten by a rattle snake and recovered after the administration of carrot seed essential oil, I decided to research which animals selected this plant in the wild and for what reason. Rattle snake bites cause internal bleeding and carrot seed essential oil had an immediate effect on the blood dripping from his nose (refer to Gunnar story below). In my search, I discovered that the North American starling selected plants from which carrot seed is extracted, perhaps 'innately' to prevent blood loss.

The starlings select aromatic plants such as *Daucus carota* (carrot seed) and *Achillea millefolia* (yarrow) amongst other complex aromatics to line their nests; they go out of their way to search for these. When scientists removed the aromatic plants from some of the nests they found that the chicks were subsequently infested with mites. When they took the experiment on a stage further and removed the leaves of the carrot seed plant, they discovered that the chicks had lower haemoglobin levels, suggesting that they were losing more blood to blood sucking mites.

The starlings, ability to detect volatile oils is most acute at the beginning of the breeding season, but not afterwards in September.[1] In my opinion this suggests that their selection of aromatic plants is innate (not learned) and is perhaps influenced by seasonal changes in hormones. By the second year, the male birds are more efficient in finding the plants as they will know where they are located.

I have since found that animals that have internal injuries generally select carrot seed, this remarkable ability to repair is thought to be due to its effect on the liver. I have consequently heard of other successful cases when treating rattle snake bites with carrot seed essential oil.

The effects of carrot seed essential oil on a dog bitten by a rattlesnake

On a hot summer's evening, Gunnar, my 12 month old German Shepherd dog, came to greet me after his usual exploration of the chaparral that surrounded our house. I was alarmed to see that he had considerable swelling to the chest and neck area, which had doubled in size. Totally unaware of the symptoms, I later found out it was a rattlesnake bite, so I called the vet.

He was rushed to the animal hospital, where he was given an anti-venom drip throughout the night. On arrival his blood platelet count was at 70.00 (a healthy dog is around 200.00). During the night while on the drip, it dropped further to 45.00. At that time of year the snakes' venom is at its worst. The following morning we were told that Gunnar had not responded to the drip and that there was little else that could be done. Internal bleeding had began so we had the option of taking him home or leaving him there. We took him home; my husband carried Gunnar into the house and laid him down on the floor. His life was draining from him; he probably only had hours left to live. As a last resort I tested him using kinesiology (muscle testing); blood had begun to trickle out of his nose: (rattlesnake bites cause their victim to die from internal bleeding). He responded to carrot seed, of which at that time I had little knowledge, other than that it had some affinity with cell repair. The muscle testing response to it was incredibly strong. I filled a gelatin capsule with the carrot seed mixed with a very small amount of base oil, and managed to get him to swallow it. The dose was larger than I would normally have given, but I knew that it was needed to stimulate life that was slipping away from him. We were amazed to see that almost simultaneously with the application, the blood coming from his nose subsided to a slow drip. I then applied some undiluted lavender oil to the bites, having previously read that Dr Jean Valnet, the pioneer of essential oil therapy, applied lavender to those bitten by snakes in the Alps.

Four hours later, the slow drip began to increase, but it was not as fast as at the onset. Again I gave another capsule of carrot seed and again the response was the same, with the blood subsiding. This went on throughout the night, at four-hourly intervals, with each treatment following the same pattern of improvement. Once he had made it through the night I was confident that he would make a full recovery. The following morning there were only traces of blood on the kitchen floor, but he was still very weak, and barely able to walk. By 6 pm he was showing good signs of recovery, with the appearance of blood only being displayed if he exerted himself. We retested Gunnar using kinesiology and this time he responded to sandalwood, but by 11 pm he began to regress slightly and he again responded to carrot seed and lavender. He was given a single capsule of carrot seed for the night, and lavender was applied to the areas that had been bitten.

The next day Gunnar had regained some of his strength and began to play with his canine companion, Roxy, although if he exerted himself, blood would again trickle from his nose. He was given booster capsules containing carrot seed for the following three days until he had no further interest in them, by which time he had made a full recovery.

aromatics and self-selection

Animal Aromatics is not aromatherapy

Animal Aromatics works on the principle of giving back to animals the medicinal, non-food range of remedies similar in their chemical make-up to those they would naturally seek and use in the wild. These include a variety of essential oils, absolutes, plant extracts, macerated oils such as comfrey, tubers from the devil's claw, clay, spirulina, rosehips and seaweed. Animal Aromatics encourages and allows the animal to guide its own treatment using its innate responses. The external application of extracts and oils is also used, but only to specific areas for the treatment of conditions such as wounds, sweet itch, mud fever, skin problems and aches and sprains. Most importantly, an animal must always be allowed to walk away from the application. If you work with these principles you are unlikely to go wrong.

'Aromatherapy' is a term that generally implies a full body massage with sweet smelling fragrances. To massage oil over an animal's body would be unnatural for the animal, and would most likely cause distress, clogging up the pores of the skin whilst attracting dirt. This method of application could easily result in an overdose due to the many hair follicles on an animal that provide a fast route into the bloodstream. In addition the animal would not be able to self-medicate its dose as it would instinctively do in the wild.

To diffuse oils into the environment would also not be a good idea and could result in an overdose. Those who have worked with essential oils and animals know that it can sometimes take only a few sniffs of an inspired odour to produce a profound reaction. This may include going into a trance, yawning or lying down and sleeping within minutes of inhalation. More than several sniffs could be too much for some animals and result in an unpleasant experience. The dosage and the frequency of a selected remedy must be guided by the animal.

Relationships between plants and mammals

Through evolution, mammals have developed a relationship with medicinal plants. Plants with antibacterial properties, for example, protect both the plant and the animal that eats it, thus guarding both species from disease. Animals requiring the plant's medicinal properties acquire a taste for them, while the plant's bitterness deters the healthy animal from eating it, thus the plant is protected from being completely consumed and the healthy animal is protected from possible plant toxins.

The complex relationship between mammals and plants has resulted in mammals developing an enzymatic physiology that has adapted to break down and neutralise most plant compounds. Such a process is not seen with many synthetic drugs, where the body has the inability to efficiently metabolise the active compounds, leading to potential toxicity or side effects.

Secondary compounds (metabolites) found in plants that can protect both the plant and the animal include:
- Providing antimicrobial agents
- Helping to heal wounds
- Assisting photo- repair
- Regulating temperature

At times of stress, most essential oil bearing plants increase their production of aromatic compounds, suggesting that they must play a valuable role in the function and survival of the plant. There is no general site of synthesis common to oil producing plants, but there are often similarities between plants of the same botanical family. What is common to most sites of essential oil synthesis is that it takes place in specialised cells or areas isolated from the rest of the plant. One reason for this may be that as they are highly concentrated they may possibly be toxic to healthy plant tissue.

Primary and secondary metabolites

Most mammals eat plants to provide them with both primary (food) and secondary (medicine) metabolites. Primary metabolites play a direct role in building the cell and take part in cellular processes. They are usually foods that provide energy and are not generally bitter to taste. Primary metabolites include carbohydrates (sugars), enzymes, amino acids, proteins, lipids and fixed oils. Secondary metabolites are highly active medicinally, they are usually bitter, and are found in many plants. Alkaloids, saponins, tannins, and essential oils are examples of secondary metabolites. They are very important for health but are too often forgotten in the diets of domestic and farm animals.

It appears that during sickness, changes in taste take place. Jane Goodall discovered this at Gombe, when she laced some bananas with antibiotics to treat the sick chimpanzees. She was concerned that the healthy chimps may also take the medicine, which would disrupt their gut micro flora. However she noticed that only the sick ones ate the bitter tasting antibiotic bananas[1].

Many people think that a greedy animal will take secondary compounds regardless of its needs, failing to understand that essential oils and medicinal plants are usually bitter and unpalatable and would not ingest them if they are not required. Secondary compounds are not generally recognised as food by an animal, they provide no obvious metabolic value; unlike primary metabolites, which mammals are likely to overindulge in regardless of their immediate needs, in order to store fat for survival in case food becomes scarce.

All plants are medicinal to varying degrees.

Animal Aromatics - is it safe?

Animal Aromatics is inherently safe, after all at one time it was the only natural medicine on this planet that was utilised for our survival and it has been employed by mammals since the dawn of time. What better testimonial for the long term use of these medicines? It is not an alternative or complementary therapy of recent years; it is the oldest therapy known to man that allows an animal to use its innate ability to select the remedies it needs and guide its dosage. It is this innate 'knowing' that is the key to Animal Aromatics.

The powerful secondary compounds found within many medicinal plants have a biological activity that can be both medicinal and toxic in nature. Whether such substances end up being toxic or medicinal in their effects has a great deal to do with dosage. Plant oils are normally taken in small quantities by an animal when it needs a plant's specific medicinal properties. Once the animal has selected its remedy, it will then guide the treatment by inhaling it, taking it orally or by rubbing a part of its body into it. When the condition has cleared or improved, the animal will normally reject aromas that were previously chosen and enjoyed.

In the wild, animals rarely poison themselves, however, captive horses have been known to poison themselves by grazing on plants of the genus *Senecio*, such as ragwort, which contain pyrrolizidine alkaloids that can cause liver damage. Interestingly though, in small doses these alkaloids have been seen to reduce the growth of cancerous tumours[1]. When an animal suffers from the effects of poisonous plants, it is usually because the ecological balance has been disrupted. Intense hunger can also force animals to eat medicinal plants that they would normally avoid; this is because plants are composed of both primary metabolites (food) and secondary metabolites (medicine) contained within them. The degree of bitterness usually determines their potency. Eating plants for hunger would not apply to essential oils, which are purely secondary metabolites extracted from the plant. In the wild when an animal is forced to eat medicinal plants it would normally seek out another remedy such as clay, to counteract these plant toxins.

Problems can also occur when animals come into contact with chemicals that their senses don't recognise. For example, a dog's passion for drinking anti-freeze is most likely because it cannot identify the chemicals and this confuses their senses.

Animals 'know'

Gorillas in the Bwindi impenetrable National Park in Uganda will suck on wood chips for several minutes before spitting them out. Sometimes, they chew on them until their gums bleed. They have also been seen breaking off pieces of wood for later use. Researchers speculated that perhaps the wood was providing some kind of medicinal benefit. A study by Cornell University observed 15 gorillas of different ages and gender as they engaged in wood-eating activities. The researchers found that the decayed wood was the source of over 95 percent of the animal's dietary sodium[2].

Plants that cause a reaction can treat that same reaction

Most essential oils have been tested for their lethal dose by administering very large amounts to a range of mammals. These results then become the guide to essential oil toxicity; unfortunately however, this data is obtained from animals that have had essential oils and plant chemicals forced upon them at doses that would never be achieved in a normal situation and there is no data that I am aware of on self-selection, such research I am sure would offer very different results. The current published data on plant extracts has warned many people away from the very plants the animal may need to restore its health.

A plant appears to only cause an adverse reaction when it is not needed

From my observations, I have seen that essential oils and plant extracts that are contraindicated for a particular condition are often selected by animals for that very same condition. It Appears that plants offer medicinal properties that help to bring the body back into balance. For example, neurotoxic oils, such as peppermint are generally selected by animals with nerve damage. Fennel is a galactagogue (stimulates milk production) yet it also has the ability to dry up milk, if suckling is taking place. Rose helps bring animals both in and out of season, depending on what is needed. This then would throw questions on standard toxicology testing on animals not needing plant chemicals. Another example of how a supposedly 'toxic' remedy may assist the very condition it is supposed to cause is when horses that are prone to sun burn select photo-reactive oils to alleviate the problem. The oils appear to rebalance skin pigmentation, however, if such remedies are not needed they can cause problems such as burning and lesions of the skin.

Oils that can cause a photo-toxic reaction, it seems can also stimulate photo repair. The answer could lie in the work of a scientist called Fritz-Albert Popp[3]. Popp worked with benzo[a]pyrene, a substance known to be carcinogenic. He found that when he exposed this compound to ultraviolet (UV) light, it absorbed the light and then re-emitted it at a different frequency. He also found that if a cell is irradiated with high intensity UV light so that 99 per cent of the cell, including it's DNA, is destroyed, it can almost entirely be repaired by illuminating the cell with the same wavelength of a very weak intensity. He subsequently linked his findings to a phenomenon called 'photo repair'. Cancer-causing substances scramble ultraviolet light and emit it at a certain wavelength (380 nanometres) and Popp discovered that photo repair works most efficiently at exactly the same wavelength but at a lower intensity. It appears that photo-reactive essential oil compounds may stimulate photo repair of dysfunctional cells by enabling them to absorb light and emit it at a different frequency. Horses with sarcoids (a cutaneous, fibroblastic tumour) normally select photo-reactive oils such as bergamot, angelica root and St. John's wort macerated oil. In many cases, the sarcoid falls off or is reabsorbed into the body. Dogs with tumours or lumps will often select bergamot.

Interestingly, a new photo-dynamic therapy is being researched in Australia that produces positive results using photo-reactive substances to treat sarcoids[4]. A group of scientists researched in vitro and in vivo evaluation of hypericin for photo-dynamic therapy of equine sarcoids[5]. In one experiment they applied hypericin to eight of the ten sarcoids on a donkey and then activated them with ultra violet light; the sarcoids reduced by 90%. Perhaps had the donkey selected the photo-reactive oil most suited to its body type, or had other oils to support bodily functions they may have completely disappeared?

Photosensitisation

Photosensitisation occurs when the skin has simultaneous contact with a photo-reactive substance (such as angelica root, bergamot and St. John's wort) and sunlight. Both factors have to be present and are dose related - the stronger the dose of photo-reactive substance and the stronger the intensity of the sunlight - the more intense the adverse skin reaction.

Typical manifestation is of a swollen, inflamed, sunburned appearance that can form into lesions, resulting in secondary bacterial infection.

Photosensitisation mainly affects grey horses, fair-skinned animals, those with lightly pigmented areas, and also animals with liver disease. In cases of liver disease, phylloerythrin, a by-product of chlorophyll is not completely removed from the circulation by the liver due to the reduction of bile, so when the chlorophyll reaches the skin it causes photosensitization.

Labrador dogs from the same household with faded pigmentation on their nose Tamara Roberts 2005

The dog with the least pigmentation was selected for treatment. Remedies were offered to him and he chose bergamot and St John's wort; both remedies are photo-reactive. He also selected spirulina (algae) and carrot macerated oil. Within four weeks, his nose was black again. The remaining three dogs that were not treated had no change to their pink noses.

During the winter months noses do fade but they should return to black in the summer months. This appears to be a condition that is caused by a reaction to light which photo-reactive oils can help bring back into balance.

Toxicity

One man's medicine is another man's poison; just as there are no intrinsically safe essential oils, there are no inherently toxic ones. Toxicity occurs solely as a result of incorrect dosage and / or inappropriate administration. Terms such as 'external', 'internal', 'safe', 'toxic' all seem to have little bearing on safety in comparison to letting an animal guide the treatment. There have been many adverse reactions with oils that have been marked as 'safe'. For example, tea tree oil applied externally has sometimes caused temporary paralysis in dogs and cats, and severe skin reactions to horses' legs. In fact, tea tree oil is not the most popular oil with animals, possibly due to its 1,8-cineole content, yet it is found in many animal aromatherapy products. The quality of the oil, and whether it was first offered to the animal to assess its response to the aroma, must also be considered as possible causes of adverse reactions.

An application that is marked 'safe for inhalation' does not mean that it always is. Conversely, an oil generally thought to be hazardous, such as great mugwort or wintergreen, is not universally so if it is needed by the animal and offered correctly.

There are a number of case reports in the scientific literature concerning serious and fatal outcomes of ingesting large quantities of essential oils, but these are usually due to accidental ingestion by young children or through deliberate misuse. Few problems are reported when essential oils are used responsibly and appropriately. It is important to respect essential oils but it is a great shame that essential oils have been denied their correct use through fear and control.

Wintergreen essential oil is a good example of a beneficial oil being avoided in therapy due to its potential toxicity. If approximately 10 drops of wintergreen oil, which contains 98% methyl salicylate, were totally absorbed into the body, the dose could be compared to taking two tablets of aspirin at 325mg each (which contains salicylate compounds). When a horse goes past a basket willow tree, *Salix caprea,* it may well try to strip it of its leaves. This is because the basket willow tree contains natural pain killing and anti-inflammatory compounds similar to those found in wintergreen.

Animals will self-select wintergreen safely and yet it is considered to be a potentially toxic essential oil and generally avoided by aromatherapists. An essential oil dilution used in aromatherapy is commonly around 2.5%, yet it is possible to buy retail products that contain 10-30% salicylate compounds, from which very few negative effects are reported.

Caution:
The main contraindication when using wintergreen is to avoid it if anticoagulant drugs such as warfarin are being taken, or if the animal is unable to metabolise salicylates (cats) or is allergic to aspirin.

A pony selects wintergreen. Caroline Ingraham 2001

A pony had been put on box rest for a year due to an injury that caused a perforated tendon. Six months into her confinement she was offered wintergreen and loved it. It was applied topically in a blend with other anti-inflammatory oils. When she received her twice daily application, she immediately relaxed, putting her ears forward. Within two weeks the tendon had repaired by 70 percent and she was off box rest shortly afterwards - five months earlier than expected.

An oil marked 'safe' causes an adverse reaction and an oil marked 'hazardous' provides relief. Caroline Ingraham

Beth is a seventeen-year-old mare with a ten-year history of severe respiratory problems, which include COPD in winter and violent asthma attacks. These symptoms had been treated with high dosages of drug therapy and a nebuliser for 5 days in 20, which kept Beth alive but barely able to walk. Eventually the vet said that there was little more that he could do and he agreed to the owner's request to try essential oils. She began with a topical application of spearmint and great mugwort, an antihistaminic essential oil considered to be hazardous. Beth also responded to an oral application of seaweed that is detoxifying.

After two weeks of taking the oils daily, Beth had improved and was free of all drugs except the nebuliser. She then turned away from the oils that she had previously chosen and selected German chamomile, a milder antihistaminic essential oil but stronger anti-inflammatory remedy than great mugwort and she also selected garlic - this was interesting as Beth was the only one among the owner's horses that had refused garlic granules in her feed (essential oils can be quite different in their chemical make up to the plants from which they are extracted). Beth was enthusiastic about garlic oil, which she took orally off and on for the following nine months. During this time Beth remained free of drugs and only needed the nebuliser occasionally. She breathed normally and moved around her paddock with ease. Her owner intended to start riding her gently the following month.

Following the success of the treatment, Beth's owner read that eucalyptus, a supposedly 'safe' essential oil, was good for the lungs. Beth was not particularly enthusiastic about it but several drops were put onto a piece of cotton wool and placed in a nosebag for her to inhale the vapours. As a result of being forced to inhale an oil without being able to guide the dosage, Beth had a violent, life threatening asthma attack. Conventional drugs had to be administered again. After two weeks she went back to her original essential oil therapy and is now free of drugs again. This shows that an oil marked as 'safe' is not necessarily so if the animal has not been able to guide the selection and dosage.

Caution: Never force an animal to inhale an aroma or apply a remedy topically that it has not selected, it will provide no benefit and may cause harm.

Secondary compounds in the feed ?

When remedies such as garlic or seaweed are added to an animal's feed, either in their dried form or as an essential oil, it is done with 'knowledge', rather than 'knowing'. Dried garlic and seaweed are possibly two of the most frequently used supplements that are put into a horse's feed. They are both secondary metabolites and are therefore medicinal - they are not food. Adding remedies to an animal's food means that the animal is forced to eat them and has no control over its individual dosage.

If a medicine is given that is not needed, it may cause an adverse reaction. Garlic acts to thin the blood, so it would be unwise to put it into the feed without allowing the animal to self-select it first. This is especially true if the animal is prone to haemorrhaging. Both too much, and too little, iodine can result in abnormal thyroid metabolism. The availability of iodine from seaweed is variable and it can provide too much, symptoms may include anxiety, weight loss and diarrhoea. Cases of iodine toxicity found in scientific journals are mostly from excessive amounts of kelp and kelp tablets in the diet (multiple times a week). On the other hand, components found in flax seeds, and raw cruciferous vegetables can counteract iodine. Goitrogens, can cause an enlarged thyroid gland, (also called a goite)r, if iodine is deficient.[13]

In one case, a horse with sensitive skin appeared to have a reaction to his sweat and consequently when worked, would sweat and lose hair around the brow band; this had been the case for several years, the hair would then re-grow white. However, when garlic was omitted from the feed, the horse no longer lost hair around this area and it did not appear to sweat up so much, further more the hair re-grew back to its normal colour.

The most popular of all secondary compounds fed as a supplement to the horse is rosehips; these become widely available throughout the countryside during the autumn months. Rosehips contain one of the richest sources of vitamin C; so it makes sense that horses are attracted to eat then in order to stock up and support the immune system and bodily function for the long winter months ahead. I have noticed that horses will consume much larger quantities in the winter than the summer, which reflects their natural availability - once again we are seeing the relationship between plants and animals. Rosehips are more readily available in the wild to the horse and more frequently selected than garlic and seaweed, however unfortunately commercial companies play a huge role in dictating an animal's needs.

Since the needs of every animal will vary according to its physical and emotional state at any given time, it makes sense to allow an animal to self-select secondary metabolites, rather than automatically adding them to the feed, leaving the animal with no choice to select for its needs. In the wild, a horse will naturally select the elements in its diet one-by-one, not all mixed together. If possible offer secondary compounds separately from the feed so that the exact amount needed can be selected. It may be that they are only required occasionally, say a couple of times a week, so offer them first to your animal even if you do add them to their feed.

Positive research
Viruses, fungi and bacteria

The uses of plant extracts are supported by up-to-date research into pharmacology, psychology and microbiology. The subtle independent nature of essential oils and their ability to penetrate the cell membrane and influence cellular metabolism accounts for much of their success. An individual cell will continuously react and interact with other cells, chemically exchanging information.

Essential oils have two things in their favour when considering their potential to enter the body and exert their effects: they are composed of lipophilic compounds (fat soluble) and they are of low molecular weight. Since the body is made up of fatty tissue these two properties give them an advantage over many synthetic drugs that are heavy in their structure and not lipophilic and thus have more difficulty accessing their required site. Most actions of essential oils against fungi and bacteria occurs at the organism's cell membrane; the components within essential oils have the ability of penetrating the organism and affecting cell processes such as cell division and cellular respiration.

Essential oils can be effective against viruses which genetically resemble the organisms that they infect and are otherwise very difficult to treat. Normally anything that damages a virus would be likely to damage the body. With regards to antiviral effects of essential oils, the mechanism is not as clear - most work shows that they are effective at the stage where the virus is in its free state - that is to say when it is not associated with the host cell. There are impressive results now recorded of the antiviral effects of essential oils, which have lead to the development of a cream used to treat herpes; the active ingredient is an extract of melissa.

An aromatogram is the most common technique used in vitro to ascertain the antimicrobial properties of essential oils. There are several methods used, the most common one being the agar plate method where cultured organisms are tested for their sensitivity to a range of essential oils and/or their components.

An example of this type of testing is summarised below with the work of Thomas Ingraham in 2006[5.] who made a comparative investigation into the antibacterial effects of a variety of essential oils and antibiotics on three strains of *Escherichia coli* bacteria.

Analysis
All three results showed that bitter almond was the most effective substance on all three strains of *Escherichia coli* with a 100% inhibition in all three cases. Tetracycline was equal to this in one of the strains. Chloramphenicol was more effective than tetracycline on another but not on the two other strains. Clove oil was the least effective out of the antibacterial agents in all three cases. The control, ethanol, had 0% inhibition in each condition tested.

Both tetracycline and chloramphenico are antibiotics. The mechanism employed by both of these substances is that of binding to the bacteria's ribosomes; inhibiting the translation stage in protein syntheses by blocking the tRNA from reaching the ribosome. This prevents the bacteria form creating structures necessary for its survival such as the protective cell wall, so ultimately stops the organism from dividing. Tetracycline is an antibiotic that is used to treat urinary tract infections, which can be caused by E.coli bacteria. Chloramphenicol on the other hand is intended for more devastating diseases such as cholera. However, this antibiotic is only administered in serious conditions as it can cause irreversible damage to bone marrow.

The study concluded that benzaldehyde, the main component found in bitter almond essential oil, to be the only effective agent from those tested against three strains of *Escherichia coli* bacteria.

Immune enhancement / cancer prevention

Another study on benzaldehyde, the main constituent of bitter almond oil, was seen to have an effect against tumours by stimulating natural killer cells, whose function is to kill both viruses and diseased cells. Mice were given an immune suppressant that reduced immune activity by 50%, but when 5mg of benzaldehyde was given in conjunction with the drug, activity remained at its normal level.[6]

Remedies tested in a laboratory could also be misleading and concluded as 'ineffective'.

Solanine is a glycoalkaloid from a species of the nightshade family. It is derived from foods such as potatoes, tomatoes; naturally occurring in the plant including the leaves, fruits and tubers.

Two chemists concluded that a low dose of solanine protected mice from being infected by salmonella bacteria, since the mice that were not given solanine died within four days of salmonella infection. Yet the solanine had absolutely no effect on bacteria in a test tube, so would not normally have been regarded as an antibacterial agent as it only works inside the body[1]. The mechanism is not fully understood, but it appears that certain essential oils may work in a similar way. The blood of solanine treated mice contained an unidentified component that helps destroy bacteria.

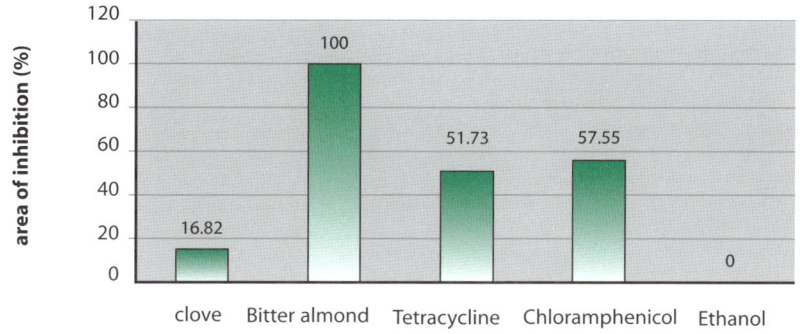

Study made by Thomas Ingraham
Antibacterial effects of a variety of essential oils and antibiotics on three strains of *Escherichia coli* bacteria

A bar chart to show the effectiveness of four substances on the inhibition of *E.coli* (strain B)

Pathways into the body

The air is full of messages
Aromatic molecular communication is not uncommon throughout the animal kingdom where messages are sent via pheromones to provide vital information on their surroundings. Essential oils may very well work in this same way by providing messages, which could perhaps explain the remarkable changes on animal behaviour in response to the aromatic remedies offered.

The volatile nature of the essential oil allows the molecules to enter the nasal chamber where they interact with chemical receptors that in turn, send information to the brain. As soon as an aroma is detected, the animal's brain will define and select needed remedies.

Olfaction

The olfactory sense cells of all vertebrates are, on the whole, surprisingly alike. The sense of smell is what guides the animal to its food, medicine, its young, and away from its enemies. It is therefore vital to the animals' survival. When an animal inhales, it directs the flow of inspired air to the region of the nasal cavity that houses the olfactory receptors. These receptors then transform the olfactory messages into nerve impulses that are sorted in the olfactory bulb and then sent to the limbic region of the brain, influencing physiological, hormonal and behavioural activity. The limbic system works with primitive responses where smell goes deeper than conscious thought or memory, and deals with instinct.

The olfactory sense area is stimulated by active sniffing that carries air deep into the nasal cavities, humidified by moist tissue, which may cause the nose to run when offering essential oils. So if your animal does not actively sniff its remedy it may very well not be needed.

Due to the highly lipophilic (fat-soluble) nature of essential oils they absorb easily and quickly into the lipid rich tissues of the brain and nervous system. Here, essential oils can stimulate, sedate or help repair nerve damage by binding with nerve cell membranes. Studies have shown that within minutes of inhalation, essential oil constituents are detectable in the blood[9]. The lighter the molecules, the faster they will be absorbed.

It is not unusual for conventional drugs to be taken intranasally, their rapid access through this route is partly due to it being devoid of stratum corneum and partly due to the rich vascular supply and large surface area of the nasal mucosa. Conventional veterinary medicine now administers certain drugs intranasally, such as vaccines for kennel cough.

Domestic dogs have an especially acute sense of smell, with the exception of breeds whose faces are flat resulting in chronic respiratory problems; the longer the nose the more efficient the sense of smell.

The intense impact aromas must have on dogs needs to be taken into consideration when offering them volatile aromatic remedies, especially those rich in momoterpenes, due to their light molecular weight. So don't put essential oils straight under a cat or dog's nose, as the animal may jump back and the oil mistakenly discarded as not needed; instead gradually offer the oil. To give some idea of how much more intense aromas are to animals I have included below the approximate numbers of sensory receptors of some species.

Humans 6 million receptors
Rabbits 50 million receptors
Sheep dogs 200 million receptors
German Shepherds 250 million receptors
Labrador's 280 million receptors
Beagles over 300 million receptors

Most mammals have a sense of smell that is millions of times more acute than our own. Bloodhounds are in a league of their own; there is a record of a hound that picked up an eight day old trail of a person, crossing busy streets, ending up at a bench where the missing person had sat briefly before boarding a bus to California. Daily, we shed forty million flakes of skin, each one supporting bacteria with charactistic odours. In one laboratory test a dog showed that it could identify a glass slide that had been touched briefly by a human fingertip six weeks previously.[8]

The use of essential oils via inhalation
Emotional / behavioural problems
Respiratory disorders
Suitable for sensitive horses
Destruction of airborne bacteria

The vomeronasal (Organ of Jacobson)

How animals screen information
Odour identification is so important to most mammals and reptiles that they have two mechanisms for detecting aromas. One is the vomeronasal organ (via the mouth) and the other is the olfactory system (via the nose).

The vomeronasal organ is found in most mammals and is used for the extra screening of inspired odours. It takes aromas directly to the limbic system (in the brain), awakening the animal's innate responses and is mainly used for detecting odours such as pheromones and aromatics - perhaps these aroma chemicals are screened in a way that would be similar to reading messages in the written word.

When horses flehmen (curl their upper lip), they are using the vomeronasal organ. Dogs and cats are not so obvious when using this organ. Dogs slightly puff their cheeks and lick their lips and nose, while cats display an opened mouth gape with shallow panting. Birds come under the category of sight animals and do not have the use of a vomeronasal organ. In humans, the vomeronasal organ seems to disappear soon after birth, its use it thought to be in the womb where recent studies have shown that the foetus has the ability to smell.

Aromatics offer more dramatic behaviour changes to animals than to humans?

Most mammals depend more heavily on their limbic system than the cortical parts of the brain compared to humans where the situation is reversed and thought takes over instinct. As the use of the limbic system gradually declined over human evolution, so the function of the vomeronsal organ became less important to us to the extent that it appears that adults no longer possess this piece of olfactory apparatus.

If the vomeronsal organ facilitates the transport of aroma messages into the limbic system causing behavioural changes, then surely the absence of such an organ will reduce the effect these aromas have on behaviour? This is the case in humans and is a probable reason to why essential oils do not have such a startling effect on our behaviour when compared with animals who do possess this organ.

The chemoreceptors of the vomeronasal organ are more specific with their sensory messages than the main olfactory nerves. Problems that occurred when the vomeronasal organ had been removed included rodents (voles) not being able to tell the difference between males and females; male prairie wolves stop urine marking their territory and were far less aggressive towards rival males; and female guinea pigs failed to recognise their offspring and made no effort to retrieve them when they wandered from their nest. These problems did not occur when olfactory nerves were severed.

The Skin

The skin acts as a barrier to most external influences. The epidermis possesses enzymes that act upon substances passing through it, which can activate or deactivate compounds such as essential oils, acting as a barrier. These enzymes can trigger the production of:

Inflammatory mediators
Hormones
Steroids

By the time a substance reaches the blood it may have changed from its original state. Terpene compounds such as 1,8-cineole disrupt the skin barrier allowing for quick penetration, and so therefore are of interest to drug researchers.

Topical use

Most topical applications in Animal Aromatics are used for the treatment of specific problems such as arthritis, aches, sprains, where there is heat, sweet-itch, mud-fever, wounds, broken skin and other similar conditions affecting the skin.

Essential oil application is normally administered in a water-based gel which allows the oils to be absorbed readily through the skin and the hair follicles and into the dermal layers; this effect is enhanced due to the lipid soluble nature of essential oils that are attracted to the body's fatty tissues. Clays are also used topically especially as a poultice, to fill cracks, applied to sarcoids and wounds and as a sun block.

Topical applications to wounds and broken skin are generally applied undiluted, these include yarrow, German chamomile, lavender, seaweed, rosehip and thyme.

Topical use of essential oils for animals include

To treat localised conditions

To treat underlying muscles / organs

To treat - wounds

To treat irritated skin

To utilise the effects of touch

Factors influencing skin absorption

Heat	Rapid absorption
Thickness of stratum corneum	Thick skin, slow absorption, thin skin; rapid absorption
Molecular structure /weight of oils	Heavier molecules take longer to penetrate the skin
Blood supply	A rich blood supply allows for rapid absorption
Presence of hair and sweat glands	Hair shafts bypass the biggest physical barrier to absorption - the the stratum corneum

Caution:

Certain essential oils can be dermal irritants. Extreme care should be taken with citrus oils, those that are photo- reactive and those rich in monoterpenes, phenols and certain aldehydes due to irritation. Essential oils administered in water can exacerbate their irritant effects.

Oral Administration

In the mouth essential oils are rapidly absorbed due to its rich vascular supply.

Sublingual (under the tongue) will have the fastest access into the blood due to it being rich in blood vessels; this is useful for infectious diseases. Buccal / surlingual (gums / top of the tongue) also results in rapid absorption into the body but not to the same extent as under the tongue (sublingual administration).

An equine needing a remedy quickly will lick certain oils with the underneath of its tongue, while others will be taken from the top of the tongue, or just inhaled.

Why not put essential oils in the feed ?

Buccal and sublingual absorption is preferred to putting the remedy in the feed (swallowed) for the following reasons:

The buccal /sublingual route is more likely to absorb essential oils unchanged by enzymes

The pH of the mouth is relatively neutral, unlike the acids in the stomach

In the feed the animal has little or no choice other than to ingest it

Caution: Certain essential oils, especially the herbal ones can cause irritation to the mucus membranes, so therefore need to be diluted in a fixed oil.

Extraction

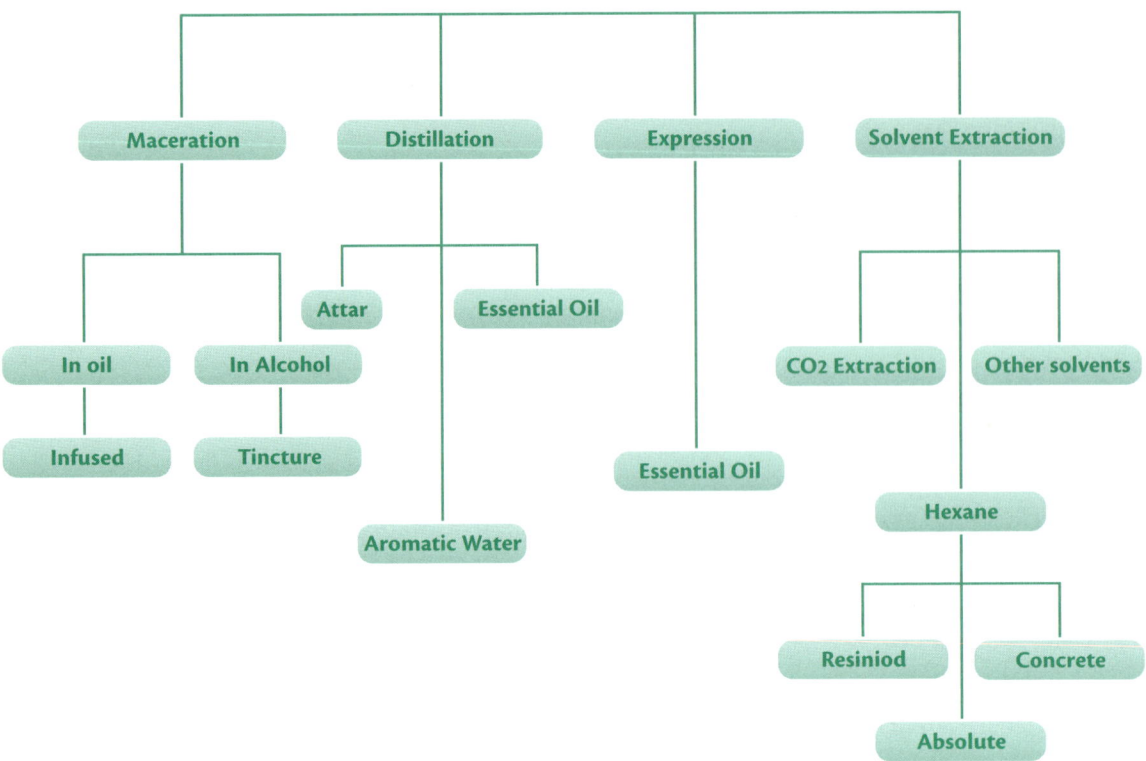

Commonly used extracts in animal aromatic medicine

Essential oils, Absolutes, Co2 extracts, Aromatic waters, Macerated oils

Essential Oils

Are volatile compounds that are obtained by distillation or expression. Essential oils are concentrated plant medicines comprised entirely of secondary metabolites.

Aromatic Waters

Are generally products of essential oil distillation. They contain traces of essential oils and other aromatic water soluble molecules not found in essential oils. Animals generally take cornflower water in larger amounts than essential oils.

Absolutes

Are plant extracts that are obtained via solvent extraction. They usually contain heavier molecules than are found in essential oils and have an aroma that is very representative of the plant used.

Examples

Rose absolute

Jasmine absolute

Violet leaf absolute

CO_2 Extracts

Are derived from solvent extraction with CO_2 acting as the solvent. This yields a product that is very true to the aroma/taste of the plant extracted. They can be very different in their composition compared to essential oils extracted from the same species.

Animals often take larger quantities of these than essential oils

Examples

Seaweed CO_2 extract

Rosehip CO_2 extract

Macerated oils (infused oils)

Are infused oils where the active plant material has been soaked/macerated in a vegetable oil such as sunflower oil. During this process, the active compounds transfer into the vegetable oil. After a given period of time, the resulting infused oil is then pressed and filtered.

Examples

St John's wort infused oil

Calendula infused oil

Animals will often take macerates in larger amounts than all other remedies, other than cornflower water.

Extraction Notes

The distillation process can produce chemical changes within the plant material. For example, plants such as German chamomile and yarrow contain no blue compounds yet during distillation they produce a substance called azulene, derived from a non-blue precursor in the plant. Azulene gives these oils their characteristic ink blue colour and is responsible for much of their anti-inflammatory and antiseptic properties. After distillation, essential oils can have quite different, and often more potent properties than the plants from which they are derived.

Essential oils are extracted from tiny secretory structures (glands) contained within herbs, flowers, seeds, fruits, wood, resins and roots of a plant, normally by distillation or a process called expression (a form of pressing) when citrus oils are involved. Absolutes are extracted with solvents and not by distillation. Thus technically they are not essential oils. Absolutes may contain minute traces of the solvent used to extract them.

Similar but different to allopathic medicine

Of all the complementary therapies, essential oils and plant extracts could be considered the most similar in structure and application to many prescription drugs, however they differ in that they work in their own specialised individual manner. A typical essential oil is an intricate mixture of chemical compounds, each of which has its own set of unique properties. The number of major constituents within an essential oil is relatively small in comparison with the number of minor constituents and trace elements. The trace elements may be present in such minute quantities that they can only be measured in parts per million. They are believed to help counteract any side effects that the major and minor constituents might produce; their full role is not as yet known.

The complex mixture of constituents and trace elements within an essential oil is impossible to reproduce synthetically. Chemical substitutes often lack the all-important trace elements and 'life force' needed for holistic healing. Their complexity and inherently variable composition lessen the chances of bacterial resistance when dealing with infection - an advantage over conventional antibiotics for which multidrug-resistant organisms are currently posing a serious risk to human and animal health.

The importance of quality

If you want to achieve the maximum healing potential, it is important to use high quality plant oils, especially as with animals they are often taken internally. As essential oils, such as rose and absolutes such as jasmine are expensive to produce, it may take 30 rose heads to make one drop of essential oil, it is not surprising that the perfumery and cosmetic worlds have succeeded in producing good imitations. In other words quality comes at a price, it is impossible to buy a cheap rose oil. Essential oils that are likely to be authentic will have the following criteria listed on the label.

- The botanical name
- The part of the plant used
- The country of origin
- The extraction process
- The batch number

Essential Oil Adulteration

It is likely that a large percentage of essential oils available have been altered in some way either prior to or after distillation.

Various ways essential oils are adulterated

Classic adulteration: mixing essential oils of more than one species in order to increase quantity and lower production cost, thus increasing profit margin. For example lavandin with lavender and sold as lavender (5-7 x more expensive than lavandin).

Isolate adulteration: involves the addition of natural isolates such as 1,8-cineole or citral to an essential oil for the same purposes as classic adulteration. Natural isolates can be added to the still along with the plant or are added after distillation.

Nature identical adulteration: mimics its organoleptic qualities by mixing isolates and chemicals together in a laboratory situation.

Addition of diluents: these are non-odorous substances that can be added to essential oils for their dilution. Common fragrance diluents include diethyl phthalate (DEP) and dipropylene glycol (DPG). Diluents are often found in oils such as frankincense, sandalwood, patchouli and rose oils.

There are also other processes that render essential oils incomplete, inferior or possibly unsuitable for aromatherapy use that cannot be strictly termed adulteration. Essential oils can be termed natural and unadulterated but supplied from old stock thus offering a less vibrant quality.

Detecting adulteration

Basic testing on organoleptic (colour, aroma, taste, viscosity) and physical characteristics (density, optical rotation, refractive index etc) is possible at reasonable costs and is within the possibility of all essential oil companies irrespective of their size. This is the first step in quality and purity analysis.

Second level analysis

The next essential step involves more in-depth but more costly testing such as Gas Chromatography/ Mass Spectrometry (GC/MS), which even though is capable of quantifying and identifying to a large extent what is in an essential oil, it cannot differentiate between natural and synthetic isolates/ adulterants nor identify enantiomeric configurations.

Advanced techniques

Recent advances in chromatography, such as chiral analysis have led to increased accuracy in detecting synthetic and natural compounds. As nature identical and natural isolate adulteration is increasingly found, this form of GC will become more commonly used. This GC is even more costly than a standard GC and few laboratories possess one at present.

Essential oil care

Degradation of essential oils and other remedies can occur with prolonged storage and poor storage conditions. Many essential oils oxidise readily so lids should always be kept firmly screwed on. Out of date essential oils may not only lose their therapeutic properties, but chemical changes can occur that may make an oil hazardous. The main degenerative factors responsible for essential oils, macerated oils and fixed oils are oxygen, heat and light. Therefore, always store oils in a cool, dark place and check the expiry dates before use.

The oils are 'living' substances and have a life span of approximately one to six years depending on the oil and its quality. Oils rich in lighter components such as monoterpenes, for example citrus essential oils, have the shortest life span and the heavier oils such as sandalwood and vetiver have the longest. If an oil has aged or oxidised its aroma will not be fresh, it may become sticky around the lid or it may lose strength in its scent. Aged oils usually undergo chemical changes.

When searching for quality I personally determine the oil generally by its aroma - it should smell so fresh that you could be sitting in the plant; it should not have the after aroma of a commercial fragrance.

Essential oils that are being used for therapeutic use should be stored in dark opaque bottles, or bottles that contain UV protection in the glass. Top quality essential oils must be used for optimum results: but their prices will make them less affordable to the general consumer and are thus usually only available through specialist suppliers as opposed to high street stores.

It is difficult to give an exact shelf life as some suppliers may already have had a particular oil in stock for some time.

The essential oil profiles in this book carry some guidelines to shelf life and can be used as a general rule.

Shelf life

Short: 6 months - 1 year
Moderate: 1 - 5 years
Long: 5 years plus

Safety notes

1. Check your animal's condition with your veterinary surgeon.
2. Never force an oil or its aroma onto an animal - it will offer no benefit. An unpleasant experience with essential oils will make the animal more suspicious of other aromas offered, resulting in problems assessing which oils are needed.
3. Check you have the correct dilution.
4. Make sure that you have read about the oils before offering them to your animal.
5. Hold the bottle firmly so that the hand covers most of the bottle. This will prevent the animal snatching the bottle and swallowing it, which has been known to happen!
6. Make sure that the undiluted oil does not touch the sensitive nostrils, especially with oils that are irritants, such as garlic and lemon.
7. If no positive results have been noticed within 48 hours, stop the oils and consult your vet or an Animal Aromatics teacher. It may be that you have not selected the appropriate oils, read the animals response correctly, or that your animal would be more suited to another form of healing.
8. As with most natural remedies, the detoxifying process can exacerbate the initial symptoms and this can last for several days. If this should happen, decrease the amount offered or frequency or stop until it clears. Consult an Animal Aromatics teacher or veterinary surgeon.
9. Avoid the eyes and genital areas, other than with sandalwood or yarrow in dilution or cornflower water.
10. Do not give a full body massage with the oils unless applied in a shampoo and washed off.
11. Do not use as an inhalation strapped onto the animal.
12. Do not apply essential oils in a base oil to the nostrils or areas where the skin is exposed to strong sunlight, otherwise sunburn may occur.
13. Make sure that the oil is not photo-toxic before applying it in bright sunlight. Check in the Essential Oil Profiles.
14. Do not use base oils on irritated skin.
15. Do not add to the feed - offer separately.
16. Never hold the animals head to offer or apply the remedies.
17. If an animal is pregnant check the Essential Oil Profile carefully before offering any oils.
18. Apply caution if you are pregnant, epileptic or suffer from a serious medical condition, in these cases do not work with unappealing aromas or those with known toxicity or other hazards.
19. Do not put bottles on ledges in the stable for the following reasons:
    The horse may get hold of them while your back is turned.
    It is easy to forget them so again there is danger of the horse ingesting the bottle or they may fall and break. Exercise extreme caution when using essential oils while the animal is on medication. If in doubt, contact your vet or an Animal Aromatics teacher, or wait until the animal has finished the medication.
    Respect all essential oils as you would over the counter medications. Keep them out of the reach of children.

a step-by-step guide to Animal Aromatics

Selecting the remedy

To select the correct remedy, the emphasis needs to be on obtaining as much information as possible so that the oil can be matched to the individual animal. This will help reduce the number of oils offered, with the objective of finding the correct combination.

Make a note of the following

Behavioural history

Has the animal been separated from a companion, (animal or person) or taken from its mother too early?
If the answer is yes to any of the above offer neroli for sadness, rose for resentment and yarrow to aid in releasing the trauma. If you are not sure about the animal's past, offer these oils anyway, they may be needed.

Has the animal experienced any unpleasant experiences or accidents in the past?
Most animals have experienced some kind of trauma even if it is not always obvious to us, which would explain why they initially select rose, yarrow and arnica. Perhaps this is to help clear and release experiences from their memory. However, they may first need cornflower water or angelica root to open them up to the healing. Traumas that happened in the past, however long ago, may need oils to release them from the 'memory cells' that harness the body and mind; which if they are not treated or released may manifest into a physical or behavioural disorder. It may be worth also offering linden blossom for past injury or abuse.

Physical problems

- History of respiratory, digestive or any other problems (refer to organ systems)
- When the current problem began
- The general condition of the animal
- Allergies (refer to allergies / organ systems)
- Excessive drinking of water (refer to kidneys / organ systems)
- Unexplainable bucking (refer to kidneys / organ systems)
- Loose stools / droppings (refer to colon / organ systems)
- The animal's feed (may not be compatible to the animal's constitution)
- Supplements / treats (may not be compatible to the animal's constitution)
- The animal's routine / recent changes (refer to behaviour / organ systems)

- Vaccinations (adverse reactions /seaweed)
- When the problem started
- Turn out / exercise
- Daily routine
- Temperament both before the onset of the condition and since
- History of veterinary treatment /medication

Caution: with the exception of antibiotics and steroids, do not offer aromatics while on conventional medicine as they may interfere with drug metabolism.

Some things to take into consideration

Illness can cause depression, so some animals may appear shut down and seem to want to give up; in these cases offer remedies to support their state of mind, such as cornflower water, angelica root, neroli, or marigold or St John's wort macerated oil. Nervous, spooky behaviour can indicate oils such as violet leaf, or it may be that remedies rich in magnesium are needed to support the nervous system, such as seaweed or spirulina. Anger may be a symptom of a variety of problems; the animal may be in pain or experiencing headaches, for this try arnica or comfrey macerated oil, peppermint essential oil or devil's claw. Resentment also often manifests as anger in which case try rose. Irritability may be due to a hormonal imbalance or food intolerance.

Select oils that mirror as many of the conditions as possible.

Example 1

A retired pony that is kept out at grass and seldom ridden and is suffering from a mild cough and slight arthritis.

Offer: Stiffness, circulation problems and coughing all point to peppermint which would also help alleviate any possible boredom.

Also offer comfrey, devil's claw, arnica for arthritis and remedies to support the immune system and the emotional body.

Example 2

An anxious dog with dry skin and a dull coat.

Offer: Roman chamomile for anxiety and skin disorders, bergamot for its balancing effect on the skin and emotions, and sandalwood for its comforting properties and its effect on dry skin. Other oils to support the emotional body may be needed as well as remedies such as rosehip, sea buckthorn, hemp and marigold, not forgetting spirulina.

Order in which to offer remedies

Below is the suggested order in which to offer remedies. It is intended as a guideline only and not as a hard fast rule, ultimately let the animal you are working with guide you. Normally they will select floral oils that work on the emotional body first, then remedies for the physical body. However, if an animal is in discomfort or pain it may address the physical problem, by selecting these remedies before those that work on the emotional body. The remedies that are heavier in their molecular structure tend to generally work more on the physical body.

Light - heavy in molecular structure

- Floral waters
- Essential oils (offer pungent oils such as garlic and peppermint last)
- CO_2 extracts such as seaweed and rosehip
- Macerated oils
- Dry or soaked remedies such as rosehips, devil's claw, spirulina and clay

Allow the animal to smell the aroma from the bottle before each application to assess how it may be needed. A remedy may be inhaled only, but if it is felt that an oral application is required, offer approximately 4 drops of the diluted essential oil on the palm of the hand, or the tip of the finger for cats and sensitive dogs. Sometimes more or less may be needed.

A few sniffs may be enough for the first day, or the animal may take a sniff, walk away and then come back for more. You may also find that an oil which is initially inhaled is licked the following day. It is not unusual for the animal to lick around the edge of the oil first before licking the oil itself, try not to rush the process. Keep re-offering the oils that have provided an interest until the animal has had enough, then re-offer the preferred remedies again, once the initial selection has been offered. If the animal has a strong reaction at the time of inhaling an oil, such as closing the eyes, lowering its head, yawning or lying down, the oil will most likely only be needed as an inhalation. After inhalation see if your animal wants a dab applied on its forehead, chest or paws. Inhalation can very often be more powerful than an oral application for behavioural responses. Work sensitively with your animal, carefully observing its body language and responses. The results will be worth the time and patience.

Offering remedies

Ideally offer remedies for behavioural problems in the late afternoon or early evening and remedies to help physical problems during the day; this appears to be the natural selection times observed for animals. However if this is not possible, offer the remedies when you can, an injured animal or one in discomfort will take their remedy at any time of day.

Animal responses are easier to read when they are in a relaxed, familiar environment. Be patient at the first session and allow the animal plenty of time to work through their thoughts and memory and process the chemical messages. It is important to ensure that the animal has freedom to walk away from the aromas and process them; horses will often munch on hay during this time. If the animal needs to be tied up or is on a lead, allow as much freedom of movement with their head as possible so that they can turn away and process the remedy.

Some animals may need a few days of rose essential oil inhalation before they feel comfortable moving on to other oils, while another animal may be ready to explore other extracts after a few minutes. Close observation will help you tell if an animal is still processing an oil. Move on to offering the next remedy when your animal appears ready and continue remembering to allow it plenty of physical and mental space. Animals will let you know when they have had enough oils for one day by 'switching off 'and showing no further interest. I used to suggest a preferred amount of oils to offer, however, I have now learned that the animal will guide you. You may find yourself offering up to 20 aromas, with each inhalation offering a chemical release, you will know when they have had enough and which oils provide the greatest reaction.

Observation is important

Observe the reactions the animal has to each remedy. Small animals may take a while before they gradually come closer. Do not compare one animal with another; every animal will respond differently.

Position the remedy approximately 15-30 cm (6-12in) from the animal's nose. Dogs and cats have a particularly acute sense of smell, so do not put the essential oil bottle immediately under their nostrils, let them come to you. Always hold the bottle very firmly when offering essential oils, horses have been known to grab the bottle from the hand and swallow it.

Sensitive animals and cats

Begin by holding the oil at a distance. You will know at what distance to hold the oil as the animal will turn the head slightly away controlling the dose if you go to close, after a while try going nearer again and see if a stronger inhalation is needed. Look for stillness and heavy eyes - you may be surprised with the results. This could be followed by yawning and various other releases.

Inhaling the aroma

Flaring the nostrils indicates that the inspired aroma message is taken to the brain. When the nostrils do not flare, the animal is taking air to the lungs only. Equines will sometimes inhale through one nostril only, this is because each nostril has a different rate of air flow. If an animal sniffs an oil, however slight, it is because the odour molecules are needed in some way. The aroma alone can be sufficient in acting as the catalyst that initiates the healing process, especially with sensitive animals. Essential oils, particularly floral ones, can cause an animal to go into a trance-like state, which enables it to access its subconscious and release negative fears and emotions. This process can take anything from 30 seconds to 2 minutes, and should not be interrupted. Oils such as rose, yarrow, arnica, neroli, angelica root and linden blossom can help access memories of trauma, so are especially likely to evoke this reaction, which is also why animals can be hesitant with these oils.

Concentrating on the aroma

Occasionally there are exceptions and the animal may not obviously flare its nostrils; so it is important to look for stillness, or blinking followed by heavy- closing eyelids and perhaps a lowering of the head or lying down (dogs), appearing deep in thought. This reaction is especially true when remedies that work on the mind are offered. Allow plenty of time when offering the aromas that you feel are needed, otherwise you may miss a much needed remedy. This is also likely to happen if you have witnessed another animal readily taking its remedies, while your animal needs time to process and respond.

Positive reactions include
- Trying to nibble at the lid or bottle
- Yawning
- Sighing / deep breaths
- Sticking the tongue out and in, licking the aroma molecules in the air - cats, dogs, sheep
- Grimacing in a way that could be mistaken for an unpleasant odour, mainly dogs, cats
- Shallow panting - mainly dogs and cats
- Puffing cheeks - mainly dogs and cats
- Blinking / heavy eyes
- Tail wagging - dogs
- Pawing the ground - horses
- Chin quivering - mainly horses
- Equines curl the upper lip (flehmen)
- Flaring nostrils
- Focusing on the aroma/stillness

Positive reactions that may be mistaken for a negative reaction: (exception of cats)
- Ears back / walking to the back of the stable
- Growling - dogs. Apply caution
- Anxious behaviour

Re-offer the remedy that stimulated any of the 'negative' responses, at the end of the session to ascertain if the response is a release or a 'no thank you'. If it is a release your animal will most likely want to inhale the aroma again. You may also want to try again the following day.

When 'trauma' oils are offered unpleasant memories may be released resulting in what appears to be a negative reaction.

This may then be followed by yawning, lowering of head and heavy eyes. Any remedy that causes a behavioural reaction is usually a positive release. No reaction means an oil is not needed. This is especially true of horses and dogs, however these reactions are a little more tricky to read with cats.

No response
If you think an oil matches the condition but the animal is not interested in it, try it again the following day, or after it has been selecting its chosen remedies for several days. It may be that the animal needs to clear behavioural or physical issues before continuing with a new remedy.

Note
Many times I have been told that the animal is not interested in the oils as it only inhaled the remedy and did not lick it - yet even slight inhalation can cause profound results, often more so for behaviour than when oils are licked, it just depends on individual needs. The key to obtaining successful results is understanding that all animals are individual and not comparing one with the other.

Example of a horse needing to work with rose essential oil to clear traumatic memories and open up before taking other needed remedies. Rebecca Mosedale 2005

After inhaling rose essential oil the horse walked to the back of the stable; his owner thought this implied that it was not needed. He showed a half hearted interest in some of the other oils but only for a few days. It was suggested that a bucket of water should be left in the stable with several drops of rose oil added to it. The following morning half the bucket had been drunk. The horse then became desperate for the remedies that he had previously no longer been interested in.

A Healing Crisis - Penny Ward 2006 Behaviour

A 7 year old 14.2 hh Connemara pony.

Originally Warrior was very aloof and nervous of people to the extent of not being caught or touched, but over time, with patience we have bonded. He has always disliked and not trusted men. He has a large amount of scar tissue (possible hernia) around his sheath, when examined the vet advised this could be indicative of a difficult castration which could have been traumatic and painful.

I had offered Warrior oils the previous year when he selected rose, yarrow, linden blossom and bergamot. He was keen for all of them for several days, before losing interest. Since then Warrior has calmed down considerably and overcome his dislike of my partner and men in general. He is a gentle kind horse that harbours no malice. Over a period of quite a short time, all of Warrior's equine companions left, apart from one on stable rest. Although he did not show any signs that this bothered him, I decided to offer him oils when his friend was collected by new owners. Warrior selected rose and yarrow again. Rose was inhaled deeply for a considerable time and yarrow was inhaled and licked. He then spent a long time inhaling linden blossom with deep breaths, using both nostrils; after which he moved to the back of his stable, where he lowered his head almost to the ground, his eyelids and lips drooped and he appeared in a trance like state. I stood for a while observing, then just as I was about to get more oils, his behaviour changed dramatically.

He started throwing his head about and swishing his tail in a violent manner. He laid his ears right back and with his neck stretched he started biting out, as if something was in front of him. Then he threw his head from side to side violently, he looked behind him at his flanks, still with his tail swishing, he lifted up his back legs one after the other as if in pain, (like a horse with colic). I felt quite frightened but I understood that something quite 'deep' was taking place. I left the stable and shut the door. Warrior started screaming. He then backed up to the side of the stable, reared up and on landing he ferociously kicked out with both hind legs at the stable wall, still screaming. It was a very powerful sight and nothing like I have ever witnessed before. Within minutes Warrior calmed and stood still with his head lowered again, after a while I went in and touched his head and stroked his neck in an offer of support. He followed me to the front of the stable and inhaled more rose. I also offered him jasmine absolute (thinking of comfort and a hug in a bottle). He spent at least 3 to 4 minutes with his nose over the oil just gently taking in the aroma, before he settled.

That weekend we went to a small, local dressage competition where a 13 year old rode him. They were both relaxed and won their event. Warrior really enjoyed his morning out. He was so content when he arrived back home and trundled off into his field. Since offering the oils Warrior has now taken to whinnying every time he sees me.

Making up remedies

Every essential oil is unique in its chemical make-up, so in order to achieve their full healing potential they cannot be classified together under the same umbrella for their dilution or application. For example, the gentle nature of German chamomile cannot be compared to the harshness of garlic essential oil. The dilution needs to reflect the oil that is being used and the condition it is being used for. Yarrow for example, which has a high chamazulene content, works most efficiently in its undiluted state on wounds and inflammation, yet for an oral application it would generally be used in a 2.5% dilution. On the other hand, garlic would not be used on the skin undiluted other than for severe infection.

Each animal will have varying needs according to its condition, age and body type. The amounts suggested are guidelines only. Animal Aromatics is a healing art treating the individual and you need to carefully study an animal's response to an oil before deciding on the dilution and base. It is important to dilute essential oils into the correct base, otherwise the efficiency of the remedy could be affected.

The animal must always be offered the aroma of each remedy before each application. Essential oils for inhalation and oral use should not be blended with other essential oils or macerates, which contain plant material. This allows the animal to guide the dosage and application of each plant oil separately as it would in the wild. Topical applications can have essential oils blended together, but they too must always be offered before each application.

Exceptions to essential oil dilutions

If the interest is slight to moderate, you will need fewer drops, but if the animal is very keen on the aroma you may want to make up a stronger remedy. This is often seen with oils such as German chamomile, yarrow, seaweed, carrot seed, violet leaf and peppermint, where the animal (usually equine) ingests 5 ml of diluted oil and still has not had enough. These animals will most likely benefit from a stronger dilution of 50%. Otherwise you may find yourself going through a lot of oils and not getting very far; an undiluted oil is much more potent, than that same amount diluted, and sometimes this is needed to heal. The animal will let you know, if it is too strong by trying to lick the remedy but not actually doing so (in this case dilute further). It is important to understand and practice this, to achieve the desired results.

Oils applied to sensitive areas such as the nostrils, must always be well diluted.

A horse with colic. Steph Gaunt 2005

Steph's horse came down with colic. In the past when he had colic, he had to have tubes inserted into his nose which was followed by surgery. On this occasion Steph decided to try essential oils before calling the vet. Her horse had not passed any droppings for 7 hours. He was offered five essential oils that normally help this condition, of which he selected peppermint. Her horse was so desperate for it, that Steph put it in a 50% dilution. He finally stopped licking it after he had taken 50mls (25mls peppermint oil). Then within fifteen minutes he passed droppings, after which all signs of colic disappeared.

Diluting oils in water

Trauma essential oils (most floral)
All 'light' oils for cats

Essential oils that are diluted in water are generally the light, floral oils that work deep inside the unconscious mind with behaviour an animal may have been born with and traumas caused by life experiences.

For example: 'Light oils for behaviour'
- Angelica root/cornflower water: to open an animal to healing
- Neroli: for loss or separation from a companion or mother
- Rose: for resentment or anger
- Frankincense: for fear

'Heavy' floral essential oils, which also work on past and present traumatic experiences such as violet leaf, sandalwood and linden blossom are usually put into a base oil as are chamazulene-rich oils (blue oils) such as yarrow.

Cats only usually inhale essential oils so their oils are normally put into water, other than the 'heavy' oils those such as spikenard and valerian which are put into a base oil.

Why use water and not base oil for all essential oil dilution?

Water is the preferred method for inhalation as essential oils generally have a density lighter than water and so float on top, allowing the aromatic molecules to escape readily from the opened bottle and vapourise into the air. This enables the animal to receive potent non-diluted aromatic messages containing information required for behavioural responses. However if an animal chooses to lick a floral oil in water, that is fine. In water, the molecular structure of an essential oil, undergoes no or little change. Water is a medium for communication, and acts as a transmitter of stored physical and vibrational energy. I have found that essential oils are more potent in water, so you need to use less. It is not crucial if the essential oil is put into a base oil opposed to water; however it is important not to put potentially irritant essential oils, such as thyme, lemon or garlic into a water base as it can cause irritation to the mucus membranes. When in doubt, put essential oils that are offered orally into base oil to lessen the risk of irritation.

Spring water is a good choice of water because it has a strong 'life force'. If it is not available, let tap water stand for at least 15 minutes before using it, so that any chemicals in it have the chance to evaporate.

Diluting oils in a base (fixed oil)
Herbal and 'heavy' essential oils

Essential oils that are likely to be taken orally are diluted in a base oil. Being lipid soluble they disperse well into vegetable oils and body tissue giving them a lower risk of irritation to the mucous membranes. The fixed oils listed in the chart are the ones most frequently selected by animals and are generally used as a base into which to blend essential oils into. I do not advise blending essential oils fixed oils such as flax, hemp and neem as, like the macerated oils, they are a potent remedy in their own right.

Base oils to dilute essential oils into and their frequency of selection

Base oils	Dog	Cat	Horse
Olive	frequent	frequent	frequent
Sunflower	frequent	frequent	frequent
Thistle	moderate	not often	frequent
Grape seed	very popular	moderate	not often

When a base oil is not appropriate
Topical application would make an animals coat sticky, attracting dirt and trap infection. An oily base would also trap heat if an animal has a skin condition especially one that is hot and inflamed. An exception would be for remedies that are applied on the belly area inbetween an animal's back legs where there is very little hair. This is generally an area used to apply yarrow in cases of urinary cystitis.

In cases of sun burn, do not apply vegetable (fixed) oils or macerated oils to the affected area as this may exacerbate the problem.

How to decide which base oil to use
The animal will show an interest in the preferred fixed oil. If unsure of which base is needed, hold one in each hand and offer them at an equal distance apart, approximately 15-30 cm (6-12 inches) from the animal's nostrils. The animal will show a greater interest in the one that is needed.

The animal is keen on an oil in the bottle, but not on the hand
It could be that the hand is changing the energy of the oil, or that the animal has simply had enough. To assess which it is, re-offer the undiluted oil in the bottle; if the animal is still keen then pour a few drops of the diluted oil onto a dish or put some on an apple (for horses). An apple is a comparatively bland food source and an essential oil would dramatically alter the taste, therefore the apple would not be eaten as food (it would taste too bitter). Otherwise try adding the essential oil or absolute to water. Or it may be that the base oil is the problem, check it to make sure that the essential oil has been diluted in a base that is suited to the animal.

Diluting oils in a gel
Gels are mainly applied to areas where hair covers the body, they allow for essential oils to pass easily through the hair follicles, absorbing into the dermal layers and finally into the blood supply. Water-based gels appear to accelerate essential oil absorption into the body. If the gel is diluted with water so that it becomes quite watery, it has the dual benefit of being able to cover a larger surface area while giving faster absorption, this can partly be explained by the oils lipophilic characteristics in a polar based substance.

Essential oils can be combined in a gel and used for the following disorders:
Skin infections / broken skin
Hot inflamed skin / itchy skin
Sprains where there is heat and inflammation

How to prepare gels

Add one heaped teaspoon of aloe vera gel to 100ml of water, then add the required essential oil(s) and shake vigorously. This will bind the aloe vera gel, water and oils together. For a looser consistency add more water until you achieve the viscosity required.

Depending on the gel, one teaspoon mixed in 50 ml of water will generally give a firm consistency suitable for isolated and small patches. If the gel is to be applied over a larger area such as the hindquarters, it needs to be quite watery - approximately 1 heaped teaspoon to 150-200 ml. Long haired animals may also need a looser gel - use your judgment to achieve the best consistency. Some gels do not let down well with water and become very watery once essential oils are added, so experiment to get the best results.

Diluting essential oils in clay

Green clay works as a medium to draw toxins out of the body and oils into the body, so it makes an effective base for poultices. Clay can be used to protect and help heal a wound or sarcoids or to draw toxins from an area.

Make the clay into a paste by mixing it with a comparatively small amount of water, gel or oil. Depending on what medium is used, the clay will give a different effect. Water and clay will be drying and drawing; oil and clay will offer a protective base and gel and clay will have less of a drying effect than water. It is advisable to try out the different mixtures on yourself to get an idea of how they feel.

To enhance the drawing properties of clay, add a few drops of seaweed extract to the clay mix. The thick paste can be applied to the affected area or spread onto a bandage and applied where needed.

Powdered clay can also be used as a wound powder, sprinkled over the wound to dry it out and clean it, or a flea powder, or tooth paste or as a bath for small caged animals and birds.

Adding essential oils to a water bowl or bucket

This application is suited to wild animals, birds, snakes and those that are prone to bite. It is also suited to herds of farm animals where individual application would not be appropriate. It can also be especially useful for sensitive horses as it will allow them to open up and heal in their own time.

Horses on box rest may also benefit from oils in a water bucket. Peppermint for example can be used as a stimulant to the circulation/central nervous system and the mind. If appropriate, several oils in individual buckets may be left in the stable, this may also help to alleviate boredom. Always make sure fresh water is also available.

Leaving the oil in a water bucket or bowl has the benefit of allowing the animal to choose the frequency of their remedy, but it lacks the personal contact between the animal and its carer.

Administration method: Top the water up with approximately 10 - 15 drops of essential oil every two or three days or as needed.

Adding oils to cloth or cotton wool

When working with dogs and cats you may want to put a few drops of their preferred essential oil onto a piece of cloth or cotton wool. This may offer comfort to animals left alone in the house. Some dogs and cats will play with their favourite scented cloth or take it to their bed.

Take your time - A visit by Dida Wells 2006

It was a freezing cold, windy wet day in early January and by the time we managed to get Ellie (a TB mare), into her stable she was ready to double barrel anyone that got near her! The first oil I offered was rose otto and Ellie was absolutely not interested. I tried neroli, geranium and lavender and got nowhere, so I offered cornflower water and this was the first aroma that she liked. She inhaled quite a lot and licked a little from her owner's hand, then she seemed to want a break. It had been a long morning, so we let her back into the field and the first thing she did when we released her was to roll again and again!

I always think of rolling in these circumstances as a stress relieving behaviour or a way to rebalance. When we approached her later on, she was already looking to see what we had to offer her and she appeared far more interested. We went back to the shelter and I offered cornflower water again, which she inhaled deeply, when she turned away from this I offered angelica root. She inhaled this for quite a while and showed a real fascination for the aroma. She didn't want to lick any but was quite thoughtful and still, which amazed her owner as she is usually fairly agitated. We gave her five minutes to think about this and she was happy to stay in the shelter while we chatted. Next I offered her some rose again and this time she was very keen. She mouthed the bottle and took around 3ml of diluted rose otto, while still wanting to inhale it. This took about 40 minutes and Ellie was very thoughtful and sleepy afterwards so we decided to leave it for the day. I left the owner with another 5ml bottle of rose and some cornflower water and we arranged to meet up again during the week.

Using a water bucket for farm animals

A bucket with seaweed added to it and another with garlic was put out for approximately 100 cattle, many of which had foot rot. The most popular of the oils was garlic. Within 6 weeks most cases of foot rot had cleared.

Applying remedies topically

Always let the animal smell a remedy before applying it topically; make sure it knows that you are about to apply it. An animal will usually let you know if it wants it by relaxing to the touch. If an oil or remedy is not wanted on a particular area the animal will turn away, look uncomfortable or growl (which in this case will not usually indicate an emotional release).

Do not hold the animals head to force it to inhale oils or force it to have remedies applied.

Blend essential oils into bases such as fixed oils, clay, aloe, water.

The poll / forehead / chest / energy field

The remedy can be offered undiluted or diluted to the poll, forehead or chest. Herbivores seem to enjoy it being applied to their forehead, often they let you know they want it applied there by holding their head still or by putting their head down when you have the remedy on your hand.

I have found that goats seem to want many of their remedies applied to their forehead. They will make this very clear by rubbing their head hard into your hand as you offer it to them.

Alternatively, gently stroke the animal's body with the remedy on your hands so that it is allowed to mingle into its energy field. This is very often suited to sensitive animals or those that need to slowly ease themselves into their healing. Avoid the eyes.

Windpipe

Oils can be applied in a gel base along the windpipe, mainly for respiratory disorders, or along the mane line in certain cases for behavioural problems. Respiratory disorders usually respond well to volatile oils applied externally, such as peppermint, eucalyptus, bay laurel and frankincense, although they can also be taken orally. Oils such as garlic and carrot seed would be more beneficial taken orally only for this condition.

If garlic or bergamot (caution photo-toxic) is being used to help prevent the spread of disease, it can be wiped along the windpipe with a sponge, in the direction of the coat, using a well diluted solution, making sure it does not touch the skin.

Paws

This is a useful application when an animal seems keen on the oil but is not sure whether to lick it. Apply a dab or two of an essential oil, either diluted or undiluted, onto one of the paws (providing the dog accepts that you do this). Leave the other paw free of oils so that when it is lying down it can turn away from the aroma if it chooses to do so.

Belly

Oils such as German chamomile, yarrow and sandalwood can be applied to the belly for disorders of the stomach, kidney and bladder. They are applied either using a base oil or gel. A gel will be cooling whereas a base oil will trap heat and be warming. If using a gel, warm it in your hands first. Apply it between the back legs to the area where there is little hair. Be careful to avoid the genitals.

Caged animals / birds

If the animal is caged make sure essential oils are not left in an enclosed area for too long, as just slight inhalation of the aroma may be all that is needed; unwanted aromatic molecules may be overbearing, resulting in an unpleasant experience to the animal. Use your judgment as to how much fresh air there is.

If you are working with wild animals where it is not possible to access the enclosure, strips of wood laced with aromatic oils or pieces of aromatic cloth attached to the enclosure can be used. Refer to the study of orang-utans and tigers for more information.

The frequency of offering the remedy?

The average length of a treatment varies between three days to two weeks. However, there may be prolonged interest in oils working on the physical body such as the macerated oils and spirulina or rosehips. Occasionally, essential oils and plant extracts such as garlic and seaweed also fall into this bracket. When working on behavioural problems oils may be needed just the once. Generally, no more than a 5-10ml bottle of essential oil is needed throughout a complete treatment. However, there will be exceptions to this as every animal will have unique and individual reactions. Some may just need the oil for inhalation, whilst others may need several bottles of their remedy. An animal may continue taking remedies intermittently for up to six months or even a year, although such cases are less frequent.

The application may vary from day to day - a moderate interest may increase to a keen one in the days to follow, or it may decrease to no interest. Sometimes oils are only needed on alternate days, or only once or twice weekly. Always let your animal guide you regarding the length of time and the remedies that are needed, as well as the mode of application. If it is not possible to offer oils on a daily basis, offer them when you can, the treatment may take a little longer but the same end result will usually be achieved.

An acute problem will usually require the remedies to be offered more frequently and sometimes with a stronger dose, however your animal will guide you with this. Generally begin by offering remedies two times daily.

A keen interest in the aroma
Offer twice daily
Offer more frequently for acute conditions; as indicated by your animal

A moderate interest
Offer once a day then offer on alternate days, or twice weekly until there is no further interest.

No interest
When an animal has no further interest in its remedies, the condition should have cleared, or greatly improved.

Summary of remedies used and dilution

Remedies used

Liquid
- Essential oils
- Absolutes
- Co2 extracts
- Fixed oils (base, vegetable))
- Macerated plant oils such as Comfrey

Dried
- Beeswax
- Chalk
- Clay
- Dead Sea mineral mud
- Dried Rosehips / Seaweed
- Spirulina
- Liquorice root powder
- Tubers from the Devils Claw

DILUTIONS		Exceptions to essential oil dilutions
Floral essential oils that work on the subconscious (trauma) Oils for cats	2 - 5 drops in 5ml water or 3 -15 drops in a bucket / bowl / or on cloth	If the animal (usually equine) wants to ingest 5ml of diluted essential oil and still has not had enough, it will most likely benefit from a stronger dilution of 50%, or even in its undiluted state providing the oil is not a mucous membrane irritant.
Herbal essential oils	5 -20 drops in a fixed oil	

Essential oils that are heavy in their molecular weight such as sandalwood and linden blossom are generally put into base oil even though they work mainly on the unconscious mind.

NB Cats generally take essential oils by inhalation, therefore they are usually put into water.

Topical application: Only select chosen essential oils that will work directly on the problem, such as:

A condition that is affecting the skin
Broken skin
Sprains where there is heat and inflammation
Infection / fungus
Histaminic reactions

Below are general guidelines that have been taken from observation – I would suggest beginning by offering the remedies in this way and let your animal guide you.

Order in which to offer the remedies
• Floral Waters
• Essential oils. Offer pungent oils such as garlic and peppermint last.
• Co 2 extracts such as seaweed and rosehip
• Macerated oils
• Dry or soaked remedies such as rosehips, devils claw, spirulina and clay

Example: 1: A horse with sarcoids selected the following:

Rose otto - (subconscious mind) - add to water
Arnica: macerated oil – (subconscious) mind
Bergamot - (mind and body) – add to a base (vegetable) oil

The remedies should be offered in the above order

Bergamot would also be added to a base such as clay or aloe vera for topical application to the scarcoid due to its photo - reactive properties.

Example 2: A dog with a skin allergy selects the following remedies

Cornflower water (subconscious mind)
Neroli (subconscious mind) - add to water
Yarrow (spirit / mind / body) - add to a base oil
German Chamomile (mind / body) - add to a base oil and a gel
Peppermint – (mainly body) – add to a base oil and a gel
Rosehips: extract (body) – water for powder, base oil for C02

The remedies for inhalation / oral should be offered in the above order

German chamomile (anti-histaminic / anti-inflammatory) and peppermint (anti-irritant / cooling) -if selected, would also be added to aloe gel and applied topically to relieve itching and inflammatory / histaminic responses (the gel may also be licked).

> **Example 3: A horse selected quite a few remedies**
>
> | p.m. late afternoon | a.m. morning |
> |---|---|
> | Rose - otto in water | (more physical / heavier molecules) |
> | Yarrow - in base oil | Marigold macerated oil- undiluted |
> | Arnica - undiluted | Comfrey macerated oil - undiluted |
> | Roman chamomile – in base oil or water | Devils claw |
> | Seaweed – in base oil (this can be offered either pm or am) | Rosehips |

Extra notes

Generally begin offering the remedies for the first time late afternoon or early evening. These usually include those that work on the emotional body, whereas the morning remedies generally work on the physical body. In acute cases, offer them straight away or as needed.

It is not necessary to clean the hand each time you offer a new remedy, but any surplus should be wiped off with a rag.

Essential oils are lipid soluble, meaning they readily absorb into oil, body fat, nerve tissue and muscle. They are not water soluble so will generally float on top of water, making their way into fats, if they become available. Therefore, if the oils are applied in an aqueous solution they will absorb more quickly into the body, than if applied topically in a base oil

Caution: Animals with a fast metabolic rate and thin animals
The remedies will be much more potent for these animals; they will consequently receive higher doses in the blood due to their lack of muscle and fatty tissue.

Caution: Animals on medication, other than antibiotics, which can enhance both the effects of the essential oils and the antibiotics.

Many of the remedies discussed in this book are highly pharmacologically active

Summary to responses

Each animal will have a slightly different reaction to the aromas, it is a matter of observing the animal and reading its response, by comparison with the other oils that have been offered. Do not compare the response with that of another animal, as a shy, sensitive animal will have a very different reaction to the oils than a boisterous, inquisitive one.

The sensitive animal

Just the flaring of the nostrils or blinking of the eyes could indicate a positive response which may produce profound results. It is possible that an animal will only work with one or two oils before opening up to others. The initial interest may be so slight that it appears not to be interested in any of the oils. Be patient and work with your animal slowly.

The traumatised animal

If you are working with an animal that will not be caught, touched or will not go near people, try putting the oils onto pieces of apple, the aroma of which will overpower the taste and so it will not be treated as food. You could also try adding the remedy to a cloth, depending on the species. Alternatively, you could place some drops of essential oil on flattish stones in favoured areas or in a water bucket (make sure there is fresh water available). This way they can come to it in their own time.

The inquisitive / unfocused animal

This type of animal will appear interested in most of the aromas but will have a short attention span for oils that are not needed and longer or focused concentration for those that are required. You may want to try vertiver or valerian to bring the animal into focus.

Negative reactions

If an animal does not appear to accept any of the plant extracts it may be that you have not found the remedy to match your animal's needs, or it might be that you are not reading his responses correctly, or that another treatment such as dentistry is needed. It is important to try to eliminate any known causes of the problem. In situations where the cause is out of your control and can not be dealt with, oils such as rose serve to help the animal's ability to cope.

Results

Significant healing is usually seen within days of an animal taking the oils; sometimes the effects can be immediate. A slight deterioration of the condition may initially appear, known as a healing crisis, where the body rids itself of toxins. Signs of a healing crisis can be: diarrhoea, mucus discharge, a cough that appears to worsen, skin eruptions, or irritable, angry behaviour. If an animal experiences such symptoms, it normally lasts for no longer than a couple of days. If symptoms persist, stop the remedies and consult a qualified animal aromatic teacher or vet.

Do not apply a remedy to an animal if it has not been selected

Try to think for a moment of an essential oil or aroma that makes you feel quite sick and heady, or one from which you quickly turn your head away in disgust. If that oil were applied to your body it would make you feel quite ill and the same applies to an animal. Never assume that an oil is needed because it worked well for another animal. Pay attention to each animal's responses and respect its instincts.

Many people find it difficult to understand that the aroma alone can be a powerful tool and so are tempted to force remedies orally. Unless an animal chooses to take its remedy, this would be an overdose and toxic to the animal.

An example of a horse selecting oils

When I started to work with Uby he was very aggressive and fearful, showing signs of deep distress and sorrow. He spent most of his time tucked up, not wanting to be noticed.

Day 1

Yarrow: mouths the bottle straight away, very keen. He takes three licks using the top and bottom of the tongue.

Peppermint: thinks first then aggressively mouths the bottle and takes seven licks, mainly using the top of the tongue, walks away licking and chewing.

Neroli: slow response, curls the lip (flehmen), thinking, smells with the right nostril, licks his lips, thinking. Takes one lick with the top of his tongue, extends neck full up into the air, sniffs with both nostrils, walks off, head down, paws the ground then trots back, sniffs with the left and right nostrils, ears twitching, head nodding. Walks in a tight circle with his head down, then from a distance he looks towards me flaring his nostrils wide. He then lowers his head to the ground and stands very still. After a while he walks, still with his head down, to see his companion. I have never seen him as relaxed as this, his eyes are closing and he is taking very long, deep breaths.

Rose absolute: short sharp sniff with the right nostril. He walks off, head down, chewing. He spends a good two to three minutes thinking, as if in a trance. He then stretches out to smell the oils at a distance, his eyes wide. Lowering his head he swings it from side to side then turns away and lays down. It looks as if he is asleep.

Day 2

Yarrow: immediately nibbles the bottle, takes one lick, then walks away. He has had enough.

Neroli: sniffs with the right nostril then walks away chewing, but does not come back for more.

Peppermint: smells from a distance then is distracted by a mare in a nearby paddock.

Rose absolute: smells with both nostrils, snorts and flares his nostrils making loud noises, eyes glaze over for a few minutes, then he is distracted.

Day 3

Yarrow: smells with both nostrils and chews, smells again with the right nostril.

Peppermint: mouthing at the bottle. He licks it four times mainly with the top of the tongue.

Neroli: a slight sniff with the left nostril.

Rose absolute: sniffs with the right nostril, then walks away with his head down low, circling and chewing.

Day 7 and 8
No further interest in any of the oils.

As Uby's interest in the oils started to wane he began to stand with a nearly normal posture and he allowed the vet to work on him for the first time. After having oils for only a week, we were able to handle him and pick out his feet without his displaying fearful, nervous behaviour. He also stopped backing off when we tried to go near his right shoulder, which we discovered was fractured.

Note from author: The oils offered are not in an order that I would normally suggest, but this order seemed to work well for this horse.

Examples of how the aroma alone can be effective

A working Labrador
Caroline Ingraham 2003

Captain belonged to a local farmer. The experience I had with him was quite extraordinary as I had never before seen inhalation alone treat a physical problem, though I have had amazing results working with inhalation and behavioural problems.

I was holding a workshop at my house and asked if Captain could be a study for the class. He had been suffering from what the vet thought to be a prostate problem, for about six months. In the days before the class, he stayed with me and each morning would cry in pain as he tried to get up, and would have to lie down again. This continued until he urinated, after which he was fine until the following morning.

When the day came to work with Captain and my students, he walked into the room smelt my box, which contains over 60 essential oils, then promptly fell to sleep under the table. He was out for the count, so I couldn't give a demonstration of self-selection. I found a wound on his leg that seemed to have been there for some time, so I decided to work with this. As he was sleeping I muscle tested him, using kinesiology. He responded to seaweed only. I decided to dilute it in an aloe vera gel, even though the gel had added no strength when muscle testing, I thought the students could then learn how to make up a remedy. As I went to apply it to his hind leg, even though he appeared barely awake, he pulled it away. To test the situation further, I tried applying the undiluted seaweed extract, which he had originally tested strongly too. He lay still while I applied it.

The following morning Captain got up with no problem. I couldn't quite believe that an unidentified inhalation from my box could have sorted out the problem. I put it down to the fact that while he was staying with me, he was not in a kennel and was let out at night to urinate, which perhaps alleviated the problem. Later the farmer told me that his kennel was always kept open.

Captain went back to the farmer and for the following eighteen months, after the initial inhalation from my box of essential oils, he was free from the excruciating pain he had been experiencing each morning. Sadly, Captain was then run over and killed by a car.

A nine year old cat suffering from stress induced reoccurring cystitis
Sam Davis 2004

Tom, an older cat that arrived at the sanctuary, had come from a home where the young child had developed severe allergies to him. Tom seemed quite friendly so I picked him up and carried him inside.

From the paperwork I learned that poor Tom had for the last two years suffered from FLUTD (Feline Lower Urinary Tract Disease). He had shown all the classic symptoms - difficulty and pain urinating, blood in his urine, urethral blockage (a life-threatening condition in male cats) and urinating in inappropriate places. Tom had also become increasingly aggressive, attacking not only his animal companions but also his human family. He was on a veterinary diet and had not responded to antibiotics so I offered him valerian, which I had with me at the time. I held the bottle well away from him but he rushed towards it sniffing frantically. I think he would have climbed inside if it were possible. I had not before witnessed a cat inhaling so much essential oil. Tom inhaled so deeply for what seemed like ages, then his nose started to drip. He looked so relaxed and started to roll around the floor in a similar way to a cat that has just had a 'catnip party' but his movements weren't crazed, they were slow and almost sensual, for the want of a better word.

When I went in to visit Tom the next day he came and sat on my lap. As I stroked him I noticed a smell of Valerian coming from his coat. (I love the smell, it reminds me of root beer!) Tom had taken in a lot of Valerian via inhalation the day before and it was being excreted through his skin. This was exciting stuff! It took three days for the aroma to totally disappear from his body - even though his only method of application was inhalation! Tom's coat became noticeably more luxurious and he remained very relaxed. Out of interest I offered him more Valerian but it was declined.

After inhaling the valerian there was no further cystitis or signs of blood in the urine. Tom stayed at the sanctuary for several months and he showed no further symptoms of FLUTD for the remainder of his time with us. He was even taken off the veterinary diet and put on normal cat food. Tom was homed successfully and he has had no further episodes of FLUTD.

A greyhound
Caroline Ingraham 2001

The greyhound had been in a rescue home for the past three years, where he was waiting to be re-homed. When I met him he was in a harness as he would break free, even from the most advanced collars if he saw a man. The greyhound selected linden blossom which he inhaled but had no desire to lick. That was all. The dog's carer then stood to one side. Moments later the greyhound lay down which was unheard of as, even in his kennel, he would only lie down to sleep. I then asked the male acupuncturist who worked at the clinic if he would offer the dog the remedy; when he approached, the greyhound jumped up in fear but then, to our surprise, he relaxed and took the remedy from him. Thirty minutes later when walking past a man sitting on a wall he went up to his leg and sniffed it.

organ systems of the body
Western and Chinese Physiology

Lungs

Associated colour: white

Breathing disorders can be recognised by coughing, an excessive production of mucus or pus, and inflammation and swelling of the airways, causing laboured breathing. Common disorders of the respiratory system include allergic reactions, viral and bacterial infections and parasite infestation. Most respiratory diseases will also need oils to support the immune system and the emotional body. You may find that one oil will achieve all these goals.

In Chinese medicine, the lungs are related to the emotions of sadness and grief and they govern the strength of the voice. The lungs influence blood vessels and circulation and are related to the large intestine; an imbalance may also affect the skin and the coat. Therefore it may also be necessary to offer oils that correspond to these areas in order to balance the lungs.

Offer for inhalation and orally

Bay laurel	infection (mainly horses)
Carrot seed	cell damage / pulmonary haemorrhage (all animals)
Eucalyptus	infection (all animals) Caution: asthma
Frankincense	anxiety / fear / calms breathing (all animals)
Garlic	infection / COPD (mainly horses)
German chamomile	antihistaminic / anti-inflammatory (all animals)
Great mugwort (blue)	potent antihistamic (not to be confused with mugwort) (dogs and cats)
Melissa	viral infections (all animals, for cats offer melissa water)
Myrrh	mucolytic / infection
Peppermint / spearmint	mucolytic / stimulating / antibacterial (all animals)
Rosehips dried	immune stimulant (mainly horses)
Rosehip extract	immune stimulant (all animals)
Sandalwood	upper respiratory tract infections (all animals)
Seaweed extract	infection / allergies / immune stimulant (all animals)
Spirulina	infection / tonic / allergies (mainly dogs and cats)
Thyme	infection (mainly horses and dogs)
Yarrow	anti-inflammatory (mainly dogs and horses)

Large intestine
Associated colour: white

The main function of the Large Intestine is to receive contents from the small intestine, absorb electrolytes, nutrients and fluids, and excrete the waste in the form of stools. It also secretes large amounts of mucus. The large intestine expels wind, clears heat and cools the blood. Blocked emotions can indicate problems with the large intestine.

In Chinese medicine, the large intestine is governed by the lungs. Refer to 'lungs'.

Offer for inhalation and orally

Carrot macerated oil	diarrhoea / liver tonic
Chamomile German	diarrhoea / colitis / anti-inflammatory (all animals)
Clay green	diarrhoea / toxins
Frankincense	diarrhoea associated with fear (all animals)
Lemongrass	stimulates the parasympathetic nervous system (all animals)
Peppermint	colon disorders / digestive stimulant (all animals)
Seaweed extract	diarrhoea / colic / draws out toxins (all animals)
Spirulina	rich in nutrients /repair / toxins (mainly dogs)
Yarrow	blocked emotions / anti-inflammatory (mainly dogs and horses)

Skin
Associated colour: white

The skin is the largest organ of the body. Its functions are to provide a protective covering, to regulate temperature (except dogs and cats that do not have the ability to sweat), to offer stimuli through the nerve endings, to supply information to the brain and to eliminate toxins.

Skin problems are most often a reflection of anxiety, allergens, hormone dysfunction or toxins in the body. The oils that the animal selects will give you an idea of the cause of the problem; for example, if carrot seed or seaweed are selected it may be that the liver needs support, or if Roman chamomile is chosen the problem could be related to anxiety.

In Chinese medicine the skin is related to the lungs as both are considered respiratory organs. A weakness of the skin such as eczema, will often be accompanied by a weakness in the lungs such as asthma.

The hoof

The hoof is modified skin. The wall, sole and frog are derived from the epidermis. Some horses have a thin hoof wall with slow growth and the wall may also crack and become brittle. In addition to having the feet trimmed regularly and not allowing the horn to become excessively dry, offer carrot seed essential oil (contains carotol which stimulates the regeneration of cells), macerated carrot (carotene), rosehips (vitamin c and biotin) and seaweed extract. Together with offering remedies orally, macerated carrot oil and rosemary applied in an aloe vera gel to the hoof wall can work miraculously to restore hooves.

Offer for inhalation, orally and in some cases topically

Aloe vera gel	cooling / healing (all animals)
Bergamot	balancing / dry irritated skin / tumours / sarcoids (all animals)
Carrot seed	cell regeneration / cracked hoofs / sarcoids (mainly dogs and horses)
Chamomile German	inflamed, broken skin / antihistaminic (mainly dogs and horses)
Chamomile Roman	anxiety-related skin disorders (mainly dogs and horses)
Chickweed macerated	most skin disorders, including allergies (especially cats and dogs)
Flax macerated	supports healthy skin and coat (all animals)
Great mugwort	potent antihistaminic / mild anti-inflammatory (horses and dogs)
Hemp macerated	supports healthy skin and coat (all animals)
Lavender	sunburn / proud flesh / tissue formation / granulation (all animals)
Marigold macerate	supports healthy skin and coat (all animals)
Peppermint	helps to numb itching / analgesic / cooling (all animals)
Rosehips	hooves / tissue regeneration / photo-reactive skin (oral) (all animals)
Sandalwood	dry flaky skin (all animals)
Sea buckthorn	sunburn protection (oral/topical) / tissue regeneration (all animals)
Seaweed extract	tumours / sarcoids / minerals to stimulate healing (all animals)
Spirulina	a key remedy for allergies (mainly dogs)
Yarrow	injured skin (mainly horses and dogs)

For sweet itch, sarcoids and other skin afflictions; refer to the appropriate section under species

Kidney and bladder

Associated colour: blue / black

Many animals, especially older ones, tend to need oils to support the kidney / bladder meridian. The main function of the kidneys is to filter toxins (mainly urea) out of the body, to maintain water and electrolyte balance and to secrete certain hormones, including those responsible for controlling red blood cell production and calcium levels in the body (vitamin D3).

Excessive thirst and urination can indicate problems to this area. If the horse displays uncharacteristic bucking while being ridden, which would put pressure on the tender kidney area, offer oils to support kidney / bladder responses. Urinary problems usually cease within a day or so of using the required oils, such as sandalwood for fear. If there no immediate improvement seek veterinary advice.

In Chinese medicine, the kidneys govern the bladder and are associated with the emotion of fear. They relate to ears, balance, car sickness, noise sensitivity and they govern hair growth and shine. If your animal is noise-sensitive or afraid of fireworks try selecting oils for the kidneys, as well as appropriate oils to support the emotional body such as valerian and vetiver. Likewise for ear problems and car sickness: try offering oils in this section below.

Offer for inhalation and orally

Arnica macerated	bruising / shock / trauma (all animals)
Carrot seed	cell repair (all animals)
Cedarwood	bruising / infection (all animals)
Dead Sea mineral mud	draws out toxins. Apply in between back legs (dogs and cats)
Immortelle / patchouli	bruising and swelling (all animals)
Juniper	detoxifying / fluid retention (mainly horses and dogs)
Lemon	breaks down stone forming material (all animals)
Sandalwood	structural / antibacterial (all animals)
Tea tree	natural antibiotic (horses and dogs)
Yarrow	anti-inflammatory / associated emotional trauma (all animals)

Heart

Associated colour: red

Disturbances to the heart could be due to emotional or circulatory problems. Generally though in Animal Aromatics, the heart corresponds to the animal's emotional state. Most animals will at some stage in their life experience emotional trauma. Very often we are not aware of the event that could have triggered a conscious or unconscious fear / behavioural problem. It may be linked to separation, jealousy or insecurity etc. Some animals also appear to be born with behavioural issues or anxieties. The memory of unpleasant experiences can often lie dormant until a related situation brings them to the surface.

In Chinese medicine, the heart houses the mind, encompassing emotions, memory, the conscious and sub-conscious and mental activity. It is related to the emotion of joy or lack of joy; it is well known that emotional pain is felt in the heart. The heart meridian governs blood and blood vessels, controls sweat and relates to mouth and tongue problems as well as chewing and biting. If your animal sweats up easily, chews, mouths or bites, consider oils for the heart. The heart's related organ is the small intestine.

To heal the spirit and the sub-conscious mind (all animals)

Angelica root	opens up to healing
Cornflower water	opens up to healing / soporific (especially dogs and horses)
Jasmine	offers feelings of comfort, security, love and self worth
Linden blossom	physical and emotional abuse / lifts heavy emotions
Neroli	loss of will / separation / sadness manifesting in the heart
Rose otto / rose absolute	past trauma and resentment
Spikenard / pink lotus	deep spiritual healing / balances chakras (especially cats)
Yarrow	wounds of the heart / emotional release (offer with rose)

Oils to heal the heart and mind / behavioural problems (all animals)

Bergamot	balances behavioural states / supports the heart
Chamomile Roman	anxiety (skin / stomach disorders)
Frankincense	fear (large intestine / lungs)
Jasmine / marjoram	aggressiveness / excessive sexual excitability / vices
Lavender	comforting
Licorice root powder	brain function
Nutmeg / vetiver	bargey / unpredictable / scattered energy
Sandalwood	fear (skin / kidneys / bladder / ears)
Valerian / vetiver	lacks focus / sedative / reassuring, 'grounding' / aggressive male dominance
Vanilla	counteracts irritability / comforting
Violet leaf / clary sage	nervous / highly strung / new home or yard / comforts the heart / vices
Ylang ylang	lack of confidence / bullying / vices / male excitability (balances)

Macerated oils (all animals)

Arnica flowers	shock / bruising of the heart
Marigold	brings comfort and joy to the heart
St. John's wort	depression / sedative

Liver and gall bladder
Associated colour: green

The liver has many functions, including detoxifying poisonous and toxic compounds, blood clotting, the metabolism of fat, the breakdown of excess protein to urea, the regulation of blood sugar levels and the production of bile. The liver has a capacity to regenerate itself if partially removed.

In Chinese medicine, the emotion related to the liver is anger, resentment and frustration. How often have you heard someone say that they were livid or green with envy ? (Green is the colour associated with the liver). The liver governs the eyes, resulting in visual disturbances when it is out of balance. For example, if a horse has a problem walking through stable doors and narrow gates, check remedies for the liver. The liver also regulates blood volume and controls cramps, spasm, tremors, contracted muscles and tendons.

Conditions that may need remedies to support the liver are: anger or resentment, poisoning, toxins from medication, adverse vaccine and food additive reactions, laminitis, impaired blood clotting or thinning, cell repair and vomiting (cats and dogs).

The organ that relates to the liver is the gall bladder. Equines do not have a gall bladder but they do have a gall bladder meridian.

Offer for inhalation and orally

Bergamot	balancing / cleansing (mainly dogs)
Carrot seed	powerful cell regenerator / stimulates repair (all animals)
Carrot macerated	tonic (dogs often select this in preference to carrot seed essential oil)
Chickweed macerated	supports liver function (mainly dogs and cats)
Clay green	draws out toxins / vomiting / diarrhoea (all animals)
Clay red	blood disorders / nourishes blood (all animals especially cows)
Lime / lemon / orange	purifying / cleansing (all animals)
Rose	anger and resentment manifesting in the liver (all animals)
Seaweed extract	draws out toxins / complex minerals (all animals)
Spirulina / wheatgrass	rich in minerals / detox (mainly dogs / cats)

Spleen and stomach

Associated colour: yellow

The main functions of the spleen are to filter blood as well as manufacture phagocytic white blood cells. It stores red blood cells and platelets and releases them into the bloodstream when required. It also acts as a blood reservoir.

The stomach, which deals with digestion can experience problems caused by anxiety, food intolerances, toxins and infection. This may lead to disorders such as colic, diarrhoea, vomiting (cats and dogs) and lack of appetite.

In Chinese medicine, the spleen governs the stomach. It is related to thought, focusing and concentrating. It controls blood and muscles and transforms food and drink into energy. A dry nose and lack of moisture in the mouth are indications of stomach or spleen deficiency. The spleen and stomach also relate to taste.

Offer for inhalation and orally

Bergamot	balancing / cleansing / antibacterial (mainly dogs and horses)
Carrot seed	lack of appetite / weight loss (all animals)
Carrot macerated	lack of appetite / weight loss (all animals)
Chamomile Roman	anxiety related disorders / spasmodic colic (all animals)
Chamomile German	inflammation, colitis (all animals)
Chickweed macerate	general tonic (mainly dogs and cats)
Clay green	detoxifying (all animals)
Clay red	nourishing
Devil's claw	disorders of the gastrointestinal tract
Fennel	digestive problems / colic (mainly horses)
Garlic / thyme	bacteria in the gut (dogs and horses)
Marigold macerate	coats the stomach / uplifting
Neroli	sadness manifesting in the stomach (all animals)
Peppermint	digestive stimulant / colic (all animals)
Seaweed extract	detoxifying / colic (all animals)
Spirulina	rich in nutrients (frequently selected by dogs)

Immune responses

The main role of the immune system is to protect the body from infection. When in balance, it is capable of clearly recognising the body's own cells from potential pathogens and instigates appropriate immune responses accordingly. There are two main types of immune protection: non specific immunity (a generalised response) and specific immunity (production of antibodies against specific substances that are recognised and remembered as pathogenic). Antibodies are produced by B-lymphocytes, a type of white blood cell which is generally manufactured in the bone marrow and spleen. Each antibody is designed to work against a particular antigen (a substance that induces an immune response such as a bacteria or a virus).

Allergies

The immune system can be greatly affected by the emotional state, therefore also offer remedies that work the mind to enhance immune responses.

An allergic reaction is an enhanced immune reaction to various triggers such as insects, medications, shampoos, feeds, pollens, hay and inhaled spores. Allergic reactions are always accompanied by inflammatory changes.

Though not proven, vaccines have been thought to be a contributing cause to some allergic conditions; such as skin disorders suffered by dogs, and post-vaccine respiratory problems experienced by some horses. Most vaccines are administered via injection into the blood stream, a route that is often not related to the original disease. Airborne diseases for example, enter the body through the nose and mouth not by injection into the blood, this can confuse the immune system, causing it to overreact, resulting in an auto-immune disorder.

Allergic conditions in horses include respiratory disorders, that cause the horse to become hypersensitive to inhaled particles in its enviroment such as spores from stable dust, hay and pollens such as rapeseed, producing an asthma type reaction. Horses also suffer greatly from allergic reactions to the skin, such as that caused by the saliva of the culicoides midge which results in sweet itch.

Dogs and cats can also experience great distress from allergic reactions to mites, house dust, pollens, food intolerances and to some medications, which can be recognised by raw irritated skin.

Immune stimulants

Bergamot	stimulates immune response - tumours (mainly dogs and horses)
Bitter almond	powerful immune stimulant / antibacterial (hydrocyanic acid removed)
Carrot Seed	stimulates the regeneration of healthy cells (mainly dogs and horses)
Garlic	antibacterial / stimulates the immune response (mainly horses)
Rosehip	rich in vitamin C (all animals)
Sea buckthorn	rich in vitamin C (all animals)
Seaweed extract	detoxifying / immune stimulant (all animals)
Spirulina	powerful immune stimulant (mainly dogs and cats)

Also refer to oils for Allergies under 'Other common problems'

Aromatics for common disorders

Where dogs, horses and cats are mentioned alongside specific oils, this should not be taken as a hard and fast rule. It is taken from preferences that the animals have generally shown when I have offered the remedies.

Allergies (most animals)

Chamomile German	anti-allergenic
Great mugwort	anti-allergenic (not often cats)
Yarrow	anti-allergenic / anti-inflammatory
Flouve	'like cures like'

Also offer remedies to support the immune system

Aggressiveness (all animals)

Jasmine	male aggressiveness / excessive sexual excitability
Marjoram (sweet)	male dominant behaviour / excessive sexual excitability
Rose	releases anger (also offer yarrow)
Valerian	male dominant behaviour
Vanilla	counteracts irritability (especially mares in season)
Vetiver	dominant behaviour
Ylang ylang	bullying / male excitability (balances)

Bacterial infections (mainly dogs and horses unless otherwise stated)

Bay Laurel	lungs / airborne
Bitter almond	broad spectrum
Garlic	lungs / wounds / skin / infection
Eucalyptus	lungs / airborne
Sandalwood	ears / eyes / uro genital (also cats)
Seaweed extract	wounds / immune stimulant (also cats)
Tea tree	broad spectrum
Thyme (carvacrol/thymol)	lungs / stomach / wounds / skin / infection
Yarrow	wounds (mainly horses and dogs)

Eye problems (all animals)

Cornflower water	eye wash / oral / inhalation
Licorice root powder	poor eye sight (oral use)
Sandalwood	dilute in water: use as wash and or oral/inhalation: Infection
Yarrow	dilute in water: use as wash and or oral/inhalation: Infection/swelling/injury

Blood disorders (all animals unless stated)

Carrot seed	helps control bleeding / cell repair
Garlic	thins blood (mainly horses)
Lemon	haemostatic (reduces bleeding) / cleansing
Lime	cleansing
Orange	cleansing
Seaweed	detoxifying
Spirulina	detoxifying (mainly dogs and cats)

Diarrhoea

Carrot macerated oil	diarrhoea / liver tonic (mainly dogs)
Chamomile German	diarrhoea / anti-inflammatory (mainly dogs and horses)
Clay green / red	diarrhoea / toxins (all animals)
Frankincense	diarrhoea associated with fear (all animals)
Seaweed	diarrhoea / draws out toxins (all animals)
Spirulina	rich in nutrients / repair / toxins (mainly dogs and cats)

Hormonal imbalance (all animals)

Basil	stimulates labour
Clary sage	nervous types (females in season)
Fennel	regulates lactation
Geranium	balancing (females)
Jasmine	balancing (male) / nurturing (female) / lactation / stimulates labour
Lemon	balancing
Licorice root	regulates female hormones
Rose	regulates hormones (mainly females)

Nerve regulators

Black pepper	aids concentration (mainly horses)
Hemp macerate	calms and restores nerve function (all animals)
Melissa	nerve repair (all animals)
Peppermint	activates nerve pathways / concentration (all animals)
Seaweed extract	magnesium to support the nervous system (all animals)
Spirulina	magnesium to support the nervous system (all animals)
St John's wort	calms and restore nerve function (caution dogs and cats)

Sedatives (all animals)

St John's wort	strong sedative (caution: dogs and cats / very potent)
Valerian	strong sedative
Vetiver	calming / focusing

Other oils may cause a sedative action by their individual effect on the emotional / physical body

Viruses (all animals)

Bay laurel	airborne viruses
Chamomile German	viruses of the nerves: Herpes virus (shingles)
Citrus oils	airborne viruses
Eucalyptus	airborne viruses
Licorice root powder	blood and nerves
Melissa	blood and nerves
St John's wort	blood and nerve antiviral (caution dogs and cats)
Tea tree	general antiviral

Wounds

Carrot seed	stimulates internal healing and cell repair (all animals)
Chamomile German	proud flesh (orally or externally - horses)
Green clay	antibacterial / drying / packing (useful for cats)
Lavender	helps to prevent scarring and proud flesh
Seaweed extract	healing / detoxifying
Yarrow	antibacterial / anti-inflammatory / emotional and physical wounds (mainly horses and dogs)

base materials

Aloe Vera
Aloe barbadensis

Uses
Damaged skin
Anti-inflammatory
Antifungal / antibacterial / antiviral

Aloe vera has been used medicinally for over 6,000 years. Although the plant resembles a cactus it is actually a member of the lily (Liliaceae) family. The sub species most commonly used to produce aloe vera gel is *Aloe barbadensis* as it is potent and cultivates well. Aloe is especially noted for its soothing and healing effects on skin afflictions and wounds[11].

Aloe vera gel is a good carrier for essential oils but it can also be effective used on its own. The aloe juice is extracted from just below the cuticle (skin) of the leaves and contains aloin, which offers purging qualities. The gel is obtained from the sap and contains vitamins and minerals, mono and polysaccharides, amino acids, enzymes, plant hormones, salicylic acids, saponins and steroids.

Aloe vera gels are normally thick and sticky and need to be let down with water. It is important to use a good quality aloe vera gel. Deep amber with 97% aloe vera whole leaf is a good choice. Less suitable gels do not let down well, especially when essential oils are added. Ultrasound gel should be avoided.

Base oils

Fixed oils ('Cold Pressed')
Fixed oils, also called base, vegetable or fatty oils, are non volatile compounds that are usually present in the seeds of plants providing a high energy source used by the plant for germination. These neutral fats and waxes are members of a large group of organic compounds called lipids. The only difference between a fat and an oil is the melting point. Fats are solid at room temperature whereas oils are liquid. Fixed oils are usually obtained by cold pressing the seeds of a plant. Good quality cold pressed fixed oils often have a cloudy appearance when refrigerated.

Grapeseed oil
Vitis vinifera

Uses

Supports the skin - connective tissue

Strengthens the wall of blood vessels

Joints / muscles and blood vessels

Vision disturbances / support the retina / cataracts

Circulation

Cancer

Lymphodema

Grapeseed oil is a great favourite with dogs, they will usually avidly select it in preference to all the other fixed oils. The dried seeds are heat pressed and the resultant oil is refined with solvents, producing a light-weight, pale green and virtually odourless oil. There are no cold pressed grapeseed oils.

It is not unusual for dogs to climb up and eat a bunch of grapes; however, a letter in the American Veterinary Medicine Association suggested that grapes and raisins can be toxic and fatal to dogs; however the seeds have a different composition from the flesh, so perhaps the problem lies in the skin. I have certainly seen no ill effects from grapeseed oil in fact I have only observed positive results. Many dogs appear to eat grapes with no ill effects. There must be an unexplored reason why a dog would be so keen on a potential poison, as this would not fit in with the principle that animals have an innate knowledge that enables them to self-select remedies, nor with my observations.

Grapeseeds derive some of their medicinal effects from a type of flavonoid called proanthocyanidin which has demonstrated antioxidant activity and is believed to play a role in the stabilization of collagen and maintenance of elastin - two critical proteins in connective tissue that support organs, joints, blood vessels and muscle.

Olive oil
Olea europaea

Uses

Mild laxative

Ulcers and gastritis

Promotes cellular growth and accelerates healing

Beneficial for the skin / coat / hair

Virgin olive oil is rich in vitamins A, B-1, B-2, C, D, K and iron. It is a good source of the anti-oxidant vitamin E and is generally selected by most animals. Olive oil is extracted from the fruit of the olive tree. Its composition is variable, depending on the olive variety, soil, climate and cultivation. Generally it comprises of oleic acid, chlorophyll and sterols. The amount of oleic acid in olive oil is about the same as that found in a mother's milk, this would not apply to refined olive oils. Olive oil aids digestion, the absorption of nutrients, and it helps to maintain healthy bones thus preventing calcium loss.

Sunflower
Helianthus annuus
Uses
To relieve constipation
Slow healing wounds
Rheumatism

The oil is obtained by cold pressing the seeds. It is generally a good all round oil to have in stock and is popular with most animals specially those that need uplifting. The main constituents of sunflower oil are polyunsaturated linoleic acid, monounsaturated oleic acid and saturated palmitic acid. The oil contains vitamins A, D and mainly E, along with the minerals calcium, potassium, iron and phosphorus. There are no known contra-indications to sunflower oil.

Safflower or thistle oil
Carthamus tinctorius
Uses
Blood purifier / stagnant blood
Diuretic
Inflammation /arthritis
Liver problems

Safflower is a member of the Asteraceae family, as is the sunflower. It is also known as American saffron or false saffron and is native to the Mediterranean. The safflower is valued for its orange/yellow flowers and for the oil contained in its seeds. It is a popular oil with most animals, especially those with joint problems and laminitis. Safflower oil is rich in linoleic acid (70%), essential fatty acids (EFAs) and vitamin E. The oil also contains a high concentration of polyunsaturates which help to provide the raw material for prostaglandins, the hormone-like substances that function in cell membranes. Prostaglandins are paracrine hormones that act as chemical messengers in the locality where they are produced.

Beeswax
Uses
Antibiotic / wounds / mud fever
Ear infections
Gastrointestinal problems
Sarcoids

Beeswax is a very popular remedy with dogs, they select it as a natural antibiotic. I have noticed that dogs with ear infections and gastrointestinal problems relating to infection (indicated by diarrhoea) frequently choose beeswax, especially with rosehip extract added. It was once employed by doctors as a protective, soothing agent to the mucus membranes in the treatment of diarrhoea and dysentery and its use for wound dressings is well known.

Beeswax is often selected as a base for topical application in the treatment of sarcoids and severe cases of mud fever where the skin is open and sore. The chemical composition of the yellow crude beeswax used in animal aromatics will vary depending on the local floral / pollen source and seasonal variants.

How to make a beeswax remedy

Gently heat 60 ml of base oil in a pan. Dogs will usually select grapeseed, however, when preparing it for the treatment of sarcoids, St John's wort is normally selected. Add approximately 4 oz of beeswax and allow it to melt. Then pour it into a glass pot and allow to cool and harden. If essential oils or rosehip / seaweed extract are to be added, do this once the oil and beeswax have been poured into the pot, while it is still hot. It is important to then put a lid on so as not to lose essential oil vapours. If the preparation is too solid, melt it down again and add more oil; if it is too liquid, melt it down and add more beeswax. The consistency is much looser when made with St. John's wort. You may need to experiment at first as different types of beeswax will have a varying viscosity. Processed commercial beeswax generally results in a more solid preparation.

Administration

Dogs will normally eat the beeswax preparation - it is not usually applied topically. however horses normally have it applied topically on sarcoids and mud fever sores but will also take it by mouth if needed.

Clay

Uses

Wound powder / poultice: especially cats

Flea powder (possibly with essential oils added)

Protective cover / essential oil carrier for sarcoids

Mineral / nutrient drink: clay absorbs toxins / poisons (especially green clay)

Clay has been used since ancient times to treat a variety of disorders in animals. A good quality clay should be fresh, light and powdery. Superior clays are dug at 40-60 meters below a riverbed, these deeper layers provide a richer mineral content. The clay is then dried in the sun to further enhance the mineral content and absorbency. Lesser quality clays are oven-dried. Clay contains magnesium, calcium, potassium, manganese, phosphorus, zinc, aluminium, silicon, copper, selenium, cobalt, and molybdenum, as well as other trace elements

Clay has a variety of uses. As a poultice it is used to absorb toxins and poisonous substances, to protect and encourage healing and to dry up warts and sarcoids. It can be used as a powder on infected weeping wounds, or in paste form as a sun block. It may also be used as a flea powder or bath, especially for smaller mammals such as rodents. Animals that paw the ground and appear to eat the dirt will often choose to take clay; mixed with a little water it can be given as a drink, offering a wealth of essential minerals.

When working with any clay products use plastic or wooden utensils, not metal.

Varieties of clay

- **Green clay:** Its absorbent and drawing properties make it excellent for use as a poultice. It is also detoxifying.
- **Red clay:** Less absorbent / drawing than green clay. Rich in iron, use for problems with bleeding or the blood.
- **White clay:** Similar to green clay but lacks some of the trace elements. This is the mildest of all the clays, so is used on sensitive skins or when made into a toothpaste. It contains a large amount of aluminium which makes it a useful healing agent and sun block. It is also useful as a flea powder as it will not coat the house with green or red!
- **Pink clay:** This is a mixture of red and white clay. It heals, disinfects and soothes and is indicated for dehydrated or delicate skin.

Water

Water can be considered a valuable base due to its ability to absorb and transmit molecular and subtle energetic / vibrational information. Movement is an integral part of water's life force and activating it enables it to transmit healing energies. Shaking the bottle to distribute the oil before each application may have the added benefit of rendering the oil more effective. The practice of using water to transmit subtle energetic information has been practiced for around 200 years in Homeopathy. In the 1990's, the French scientist, Jacques Benveniste, controversially demonstrated how water stores information in its 'memory'. He showed that molecules of other substances use water as a medium for communication, and that water acts as a transmitter of stored physical and vibrational energy[12].

Vitold Bakhir, a Russian scientist, carried out some simple experiments with the water. In one experiment he placed some water in a Petri dish, put a glass plate onto it and placed another dish on top of the plate with a closed phial of 1% sodium chloride in it. The next day he froze the water in the Petri dish, and analysed the resulting crystals. They contained sodium chloride which had transferred through the glass from one sample to another. Since the body is made up of 75% water, floral essential oils would then be amplified to their potential in this medium.

It is important to try to use fresh natural water when making preparations. Spring water is a good choice, but if this is not available you should let tap water stand for at least 15 minutes before using it, so that any chemicals in it evaporate.

minerals, algae & plant extracts

algae: spirulina
Spirulina maxima

Uses (selected mainly by dogs, birds, fish and sometimes cats)

Run down, ageing and growing dogs
Birds needing extra nutrition
Allergies: spirulina is the most important remedy for skin allergies
Encourages healthy intestinal flora, reducing the risk of *Candida albicans* and pathogens such as *Escherichia coli*
Cancer / radioactivity
Immune function / viruses
Hyperthyroid cats
Birds experiencing poor egg laying

When spirulina is selected, it appears to have the remarkable ability to reverse the course of much disease and discomfort, this is especially true for many dogs, where it plays a vital role in their well-being. In the wild most dogs would readily be able to find algae in their drinking water; if this is unavailable to domestic dogs, it is important to bring such secondary compounds back into their life. Spirulina's effects can be astonishing, especially for dogs with skin and joint disorders, offering rapid improvement for even the most severe cases. Spirulina is also of great benefit to growing and older dogs; it is often noticed that within days of taking it, the coat becomes healthy and shiny. I highly recommend that all dog owners try offering spirulina, although not all dogs will select it, a large percentage will. Cats will usually choose seaweed extract in preference to spirulina, except hyperthyroid cats that will lick spirulina off a finger or saucer. Not many horses select spirulina, possibly because it is high in protein and thus is not suited to their diet.

Clinical trials have shown that spirulina can help stimulate the immune system of some birds and in my experience they frequently select it, especially parrots and chicken. In general, birds do not show symptoms of disease or distress until they become extremely ill, so a good practice may be to offer them spirulina on a regular basis.

Spirulina is a microscopic, blue-green algae. It is one of the first life forms and has lived for over 3.6 billion years, consequently its DNA is highly evolved. It can be found in fresh water, tropical springs and salt water. The majority of spirulina is harvested in California and Hawaii, where it is washed through a fine screen mesh and then dried at low temperatures to make a powder.

Spirulina is the richest and most easily digested form of protein on the planet. It should not be confused with algae such as chlorella, where the cell walls are made up of indigestible cellulose. Spirulina contains a balance of nutrients that make it virtually a 'whole food' capable of sustaining life. Its concentrated vitamins, minerals and other valuable nutrients are readily absorbed by the body. It also contains high amounts of beta carotene, anti-oxidants and iron and is a source of essential amino acids, carbohydrates, enzymes and essential fatty acids, vitamin B complex and vitamins C and E. It is reported that plants do not contain vitamin B12 yet it can be found in spirulina. The dark green colour of spirulina is derived from carotenoids, chlorophyll (a blood purifier) and phycocyanin (a blue pigment) which is a protein that is known to inhibit cancer.

Studies have suggested that spirulina enhances cell nucleus enzyme activity and repairs copying errors that can occur during DNA synthesis. This makes it a valuable treatment for certain cancers. Children affected by Chernobyl radiation that were given spirulina had a 50% reduction of radioactive levels in their urine in just 20 days[2]. Spirulina supports the immune system raising levels of three cytokines. It has the ability to generate new blood cells and stimulate T-helper cell activity which helps fight diseased cells. This stimulation has the added bonus of producing T-memory cells. These white blood cells last far longer in the bloodstream than the T-helper cells and provide a long term defence against infection. Studies have shown that spirulina inhibits viral replication and exhibits enhanced activity in bone marrow, stem cells and macrophages, as well as greater function in the spleen and thymus glands[1]. Its effect on bone marrow is possibly due to phycocyanin which gives it its dark blue-green colour. Chinese scientists found that phycocyanin stimulates hematopoiesis (the formation of blood), emulating the effect of the hormone erythropoietin produced by healthy kidneys, which regulates bone marrow stem cell production of red blood cells.

Spirulina should not be confused with other blue-green algae such as *Aphanizomenon flos aquae* from Oregon as this algae has been shown to be toxic. The micro algae, chorella holds many nutrients but does not have spirulinas' immune stimulating properties. Spirulina has no known side effects.

Administration method

Dogs: Put approximately 1 tsp - 1 tbsp in a bowl, add a small amount of water to make it into a watery paste (do not use metal implements). If added to a bowl of water, the dog may want to lick it from the palm of your hand before taking it from the bowl, other dogs prefer the powder, however a watery paste is usually preferred. Experiment to see which is most suited to the animal you are working with. Fresh water should also be available.

Cats: dip finger into the spirulina powder and offer to the cat.

Birds: sprinkle into a water bowl or dry onto the ground for pecking. Make sure fresh water is also available.

Note: If spirulina is added to water, it will usually only last for a day or two depending on the room temperature. It will turn blue when it deteriorates.

> **A chicken with no vitality**
>
> Veterinary nurse Jenny Ward arrived at one of my workshops with a 'portable farm'. This included a chicken that lacked vitality and energy. The eggs she laid had weak shells and she looked like she might die soon. I muscle tested a feather using kinesiology and she responded to geranium essential oil and spirulina. I sprinkled the spirulina on the ground which she eagerly pecked at, then put a few drops of geranium in a dish of water, which she went up to several times. Fresh air and water were also available. Within minutes she flopped to the ground so I quickly removed the geranium. To my relief Jenny reassured me that this chicken did this when she relaxed! Within days she was laying perfect eggs and became the healthiest of all the chickens.

Aromatic waters

Aromatic waters are generally superior to hydrolates and floral waters, which are mainly the by-products of large-scale steam essential oil distillation. Aromatic waters are primary products of a specific, prolonged and gentle distillation from which an extensive range of herbal extracts can be used. Quality aromatic waters are produced by totally immersing the plant into spring water, which is then gently brought to the boil. The steam that rises carries both the essential oil and water-soluble volatiles from the plant, which disperse and dissolve in the water respectively. They form vibrational remedies where the water is imprinted with the signature of the plant and where traces of essential oils and the whole plant are present. Aromatic waters are especially useful for cats, birds and reptiles. However cornflower water has shown itself to be a valuable remedy with all animals.

Cornflower water
Centaurea cyanus

Uses

Opens animal to healing

Eye problems

After operations

Cornflower aromatic water is especially popular with dogs but also frequently selected by horses and inhaled (sometimes licked) by cats. Since cornflowers are renowned for their therapeutic effectiveness with eye problems, they could then be attributed to opening the inner (third) eye, which is perhaps why animals select this remedy if they are 'shut down'.

Offer cornflower water to animals that show no or little interest in the remedies that you have selected; it is very likely that your animal will then go on to taking the plant extracts it requires. Animals also often select cornflower water after surgery, perhaps for its soporific effect.

Aromatic waters do not need to be diluted.

Dosage guide

Daily dose: no limit

Offer 1-2 times daily or as needed

Dried remedies

Catnip flowers
Nepeta cataria

The herb has a minty odour and is a member of the *Lamiaceae* family to which mint also belongs. Catnip is a great favourite with both domestic and large cats. It is offered not as an essential oil but as the dried flowering herb (make sure you have the flowers opposed to the whole plant as they are preferred). Most cats really enjoy rolling in the dried flowers which is how they would behave in the wild. About 70% of domestic cats love catnip, the percentage among wild cats is unknown.

When cats encounter catnip they chew it, rub against it and roll in it to release components such as nepetalactone which causes them to stare, leap, shake their heads and occasionally become aggressive. The euphoric effects usually last between 10-15 minutes. Cats do not appear to overdose on it and walk away when they have had enough. I am sure that most indoor cats would really appreciate this herb being offered to them not only for its effects on the mind but it also brings some of the outside world into the house providing added stimulation. Appropriate house plants are also a good idea.

When catnip is inhaled it produces stimulating effects but when chewed it sedates - a good example of the dual action of plants. For genetic reasons some cats respond to catnip and some don't, it also seems to be selected more frequently by cats of a reproductive age.

Responders have a gene that enables them to detect the active ingredient nepetalactone, a terpenoid. Nepetalactone mimics a natural pheromone found in male cat urine, which is thought to stimulate sexual reaction. Nepetalactone is a powerful insect repellent, even deterring cockroaches[3].

Application

Place the dried flowering herb on a towel or an empty litter tray and allow the cat to play / roll in it; or bring fresh catnip plants into the house.

Chalk

Chalk developed 60 - 90 million years ago. It is by definition, a form of calcium carbonate and has been formed over time by the accumulation and piling up of dead micro-organisms such as the shells of crustaceans.

It is only recently that I have begun working with chalk, offering it to animals for self selection. I have found that those which select it are mainly dogs with joint and hip problems; they appear to take comparatively large amounts of chalk when it is mixed with a fixed oil, horses on the other hand occasionally will take a small amount in a watery paste if they have joint or bone problems.

Dogs will not usually select chalk unless they are offered rosehips, which are full of vitamin C that is needed for the absorption of calcium which is found in chalk. It is fascinating to watch this self-selection process where the animals instinctively 'know' what they require.

Beau, a dog that joined us in an aromatics class, had degenerative hip dysphasia. On one of the days I decided to offer him chalk, which he was not interested in at all, until after he took rosehip extract. The chalk was favoured even more when I mixed it with a fixed oil. With this combination, Beau could not seem to get enough of making sure he had licked every last bit, after which he appeared to be in a state of deep relaxation. Maybe it eased some discomfort as he then slept for most of that afternoon.

Most[3] of the body's calcium is stored in the bones, but calcium is also found in cells (particularly muscle cells) and in the blood. Calcium is essential to muscle contraction and to the normal functioning of many enzymes. It is necessary for the formation of bone and teeth, for blood clotting, and for normal heart rhythm. Calcium moves out of the bones into the bloodstream as needed to maintain a steady level of calcium in the blood. However, mobilising too much calcium from the bones weakens them and can lead to osteoporosis. In hypocalcemia, the level of calcium in the blood is too low[4]. The chalk described in this book is used in powdered form.

Devil's claw
Harpagophytum procumbens

Uses
Arthritis
Pain: muscular / tendon / ligament
Headache
Inflammation
Gastrointestinal problems

Devil's claw is predominately selected by herbivores. It is one of the most useful remedies to offer a horse to assess possible pain, ranging from muscular to nerve pain. It is a natural pain killer and although not suited to all horses it does give some indication as to what is needed.

Devil's claw addresses musculo-skeletal problems. The main active ingredients responsible for its effectiveness are harpagoside and beta-sitosterol, which possess strong anti-inflammatory properties, helping joint, ligament and tendon problems. The whole devil's claw tuber has been found to be superior in action to just isolated harpagoside. This would indicate that the other components and trace elements in devil's claw also play an important role[5].

Devil's claw's anti-inflammatory and analgesic effects are similar in nature to phenylbutazone (Bute). Due to its bitter properties, devil's claw also stimulates the digestion, thus making it highly effective for disorders of the gastrointestinal tract. Sometimes horses will select marigold macerate simultaneously when taking devils claw, which supports the stomach, either it is because the remedy is selected for the stomach or for its protection to the stomach. Recent research has also confirmed its use as an immune-stimulant.

The part of the plant used is the tuber. It is important to offer whole slices or chunks of the tuber as the plant's effectiveness relies on its properties being absorbed though the buccal and sublingual membranes in the mouth, which are released as the animal chews it. Once swallowed and in the stomach, acids impair its effectiveness. Do not confuse the tubers with the liquid preparation of devil's claw which has had the chemical composition altered, thereby making it difficult for the animal to recognise or self-select correctly.

Administration method
Offer half a slice to 4-6 handfuls daily (more if needed). If a horse is on bute, it will take less devil's claw. You will notice that as you cut back the bute, your horse will select more devil's claw. Even though devil's claw is mainly selected by herbivores, dogs have also been known to chew the tubers when they are needed.

Caution: do not offer to mares in foal as devil's claw is a possible uterine muscle stimulant.

If a horse is taking large quantities of devil's claw (six handfuls) over a prolonged time (more than a week) they will also often select grapes or marigold macerated oil. This interest appears to decrease with lesser amounts of devil's claw. Perhaps the grapes and marigold act to enhance the properties of devil's claw or perhaps they are counteracting any possible side effects.

Licorice root (powder)
Glycyrrhiza glabra

I have recently introduced powdered licorice root into my work and it is proving to be popular with horses, especially when let down a little with water. I have not yet offered it to many dogs so can not write about my experiences.

Medicinally licorice root contains chemicals similar to human adrenal hormones and it is used to regulate female hormones. It can stimulate higher levels of adrenocorticosteriods and estrogen. Licorice has an anti-inflammatory effect that mimics cortisone in the body, but without the side effects of steroid drugs. In studies of cough suppression medicines, licorice root was as effective as codeine, a narcotic drug often added to commercial cough remedies[6].

As an anti-hepatoxic remedy; licorice is effective in the treatment of chronic hepatitis, for which it has been widely used in Japan. Much of the liver-orientated research has focused upon the triterpene glycyrrhizin that inhibits hepatocyte injury[7,8]. Antibody production is enhanced by glycyrrhizin, possibly through the production of interleukin. Glycyrrhizin also inhibits the growth of several DNA and RNA viruses, inactivating *Herpes simplex* virus[8]. Licorice is used in allopathic medicine as a treatment for peptic ulceration, and can be used in the relief of abdominal colic. It nourishes the brain, increasing cranial and cerebrospinal fluid and improves complexion, hair, and vision[9].

If licorice is not needed by the body it will cause it to excrete more potassium and retain sodium leading to water retention and elevated blood pressure, however if it is selected it can provide very positive results.

Rosehips-dried fruit, powder and extract CO_2
Rosa canina

Uses
Supports immune function
Scouring
Astringent
Poor hoof condition
Cell regeneration / scar tissue

Also known as dog rose, dried rosehips (fruit) in my observation are a horses' favourite supplement. Owners will often find that their horses will try and mug them for this sought after secondary compound! I have noticed that they seem more desperate for rosehips in the winter months, sometimes taking up to 500 g at a time. This would fit in with their natural selection as it would be at this time of year that rosehips would be available to the horse, supporting their immune system for the coming winter months. Dog rose, with its sweet fragrance grows everywhere in the wild during the summer months, then in autumn the fruit becomes available.

In the wild, rosehips are more readily available to the horse than compounds such as garlic and seaweed. Within days of a horse taking rosehips, most owners notice a shinier coat and greater alertness. The biotin content is responsible for encouraging strong healthy hooves.

Dogs and cats occasionally select soaked rosehips, benefiting from the juice. Sometimes dogs will crunch and eat the dried rosehips, however dogs and cats usually prefer the CO_2 or the powdered extract. In most cases I will refer to them both as rosehip extract in this book.

In its powdered form it can be mixed with a base oil or water for dogs, or in its powdered form, licked off the finger by cats. Horses tend to prefer whole dried rosehips.

Rosehips are one of the richest sources of vitamin C available, offering valuable support to immune function. It is a general tonic and supports the skin and coat, giving it a healthy appearance. Rosehips also contain vitamins A and K, thiamine, niacin, riboflavin and volatile oil. Vitamin A is known for its cell regenerating and restorative properties. Together with high levels of linoleic and linolenic fatty acids rosehips help to reduce scar tissue and break down hard fibres, encouraging skin regeneration; while possibly producing greater amounts of collagen, giving a smooth appearance to the skin. Beta carotene found in rosehips has been found to be valuable in protecting against the effects of sunburn both orally and topically. Rosehips can also help with scarring.

Rosehip CO_2 fruit extract (the one I write about) has a different composition to the rosehip CO_2 seed that is commonly available at retail outlets.

Dosage guide
Horses: daily dose: offer soaked or dry (generally dry is preferred). Up to approximately 300g per day (sometimes 500g is selected).

Dogs: Offer either dried or soaked. Usually the powdered dried rosehips mixed into a paste with a fixed oil is preferred or alternatively the CO_2 fruit extract.

Cats: Offer the powdered form from the finger tip or add to water or make it into watery paste. It will be a matter of assessing how your cat prefers it. Make sure fresh water is also available.

Wheat Grass (powder)
Agropyron species

Wheatgrass is made from the shoots of grasses of the *Agropyron* genus, a relative of wheat. It has a broad effectiveness, but its three most therapeutic roles are: blood purification, liver detoxification, and colon cleansing. Grasses are a complete life sustaining food and are the primary food for grazing animals.

Grasses are a wonderfully balanced source of nutrients and an excellent source for all minerals. Wheatgrass is especially high in calcium, magnesium, manganese, phosphorus and potassium, as well as trace minerals such as zinc and selenium. All are important for cardiovascular function and immune function. In the B-vitamin department, grass has them all and is a vegetable source of vitamin B12. Grass includes at least 20 amino acids

Grasses, along with Alfalfa and Algae, are the richest source of chlorophyll on the planet. Chlorophyll is often referred to as 'concentrated sun power'; it raises the basic nitrogen exchange and is therefore a good tonic. One of the reasons that chlorophyll is so effective in the treatment of disorders of the blood and liver is its similarity to Haemin. Haemin is part of 'haemoglobin', the protein portion of red blood cells that carries oxygen. The primary distinction is that chlorophyll is bound by an atom of magnesium and haemin is bound by iron. Experiments have proven that severely anaemic rabbits make a rapid return to a normal blood count once chlorophyll is administered[8].

What are Beta - Carotenes

Chemically beta - carotene is a terpene derived from a group of organic chemicals known as carotenes or carotenoids. The name 'carotene' is derived from the Latin name for carrot. It gives the rich dark green and orange/yellow colours to fruits and vegetables, along with another group of natural chemicals called flavonoids. When leaves lose their chlorophyll in the autumn, carotene is one of the colours left in the leaf. Its pigment is important for photosynthesis and it converts the light energy it absorbs to chlorophyll.

Carotenes are converted into vitamin A, a nutrient vital to growth and development. They boost the immune system and are powerful anti-oxidants, giving protection against heart disease and certain cancers. The body will only convert as much vitamin A from beta - carotene as it needs. This makes beta carotene a safe source of vitamin A as, if the amount of vitamin A exceeds the bodies needs, it can be toxic. Required amounts of beta carotene appear to decrease sensitivity to the sun, deficiencies can cause connective-tissue disorders, characterised by hardened skin.

Recent findings indicate that high-dose, beta carotene supplements may actually do more harm than good, possibly increasing rather than decreasing the number of cell-damaging, free - radicals in the body. This is another example of adverse reactions to secondary compounds that are not needed, which is why it is important to let your animal guide you as to how much it needs.

fatty oils

Macerated oils

Macerated oils are very popular with dogs but are selected by cats and horses when needed. They are made by a traditional process of cold infusing fresh, organically grown herbs, such as comfrey, marigold and arnica flowers, usually in organic cold pressed sunflower or olive oil. After approximately six weeks of soaking in the fixed oil, the plant material is pressed and strained, and the resulting oil is what is known as a macerate or macerated / infused oil.

Macerated oils retain many of the beneficial properties of the plant. It is important to keep both macerated and fixed oils in a cool, dark place as rancidity through oxidation is the most common form of degeneration. Their life span is variable according to species used but they have a shelf life inferior to that of essential oils (between 4 months and one year) If the oil becomes rancid, the lid will become sticky and it will smell rancid.

What are Essential Fatty Acids (EFAs)?

Sometimes known as vitamin F, EFAs cannot be manufactured by the body, so they need to be offered to the animal. This can be done by offering organic vegetable oils (fixed oils). EFAs make up part of the lipid layer and help to maintain the suppleness and elasticity of skin, their deficiency may result in the skin losing moisture and in skin disorders.

EFAs are also necessary for the normal functioning of the reproductive and endocrine systems and the breaking up of cholesterol deposits on arterial walls. There are two groups, omega-3 and omega-6, each having a different function. A polyunsaturated fatty acid is essential in the diet for growth, maintenance and functioning of the body. Fatty acids help maintain cell structure and are components of nerve cells and cell membranes.

Frequency of selected macerated oils

Macerated oil	Dog	Cat	Horse
Comfrey	frequent	not often	frequent
Marigold	frequent	frequent	frequent
Chickweed	frequent	frequent	occasionally
Carrot	frequent	not often	occasionally
Linden blossom	frequent	frequent	not often
Arnica	caution	inhalation	frequent
St John's wort	caution	inhalation	occasionally

Arnica flowers
Arnica montana

Uses
Shock
Emotional and physical bruising
Muscular pain, arthritis, inflammation
Immune system stimulant

Arnica is native to the mountainous regions of Europe but not found in Britain. Preparations are made from the flowers which contain sesquiterpene lactones, flavonoids, volatile oil short-chain fatty acids, phenolic acids, coumarins and alkaloids.

Animals that have experienced any kind of shock (present or past) or those that have been emotionally or physically bruised will often select arnica. Its anti-inflammatory properties help with muscle pain and painful swellings, making it a useful remedy for conditions such as arthritis and muscular aches. Recent studies have found that arnica also supports the immune system by stimulating the production of white blood cells[11].

Watch a dog carefully if it selects arnica and only offer a very small amount at first; it may appear to choke for a few seconds after taking its initial dose, which could be a form of healing crisis. However, should this happen more than once stop offering the remedy and contact an Animal Aromatic teacher or vet. Otherwise once the dog has 'recovered' the dosage can then be gradually increased to 1-2 tablespoons daily.

Caution: Arnica flowers contain helenalin, a toxic sesquiterpene lactone. In the unlikely event of an overdose, symptoms include dizziness, diarrhoea, trembling and an increased heart rate. For this reason, its use in oral applications is discouraged as a rule.

In my own experience with animals, their selection and ingestion of macerated arnica oil (even over several months) has not resulted in any adverse side effects. Instead it has brought profound healing and well-being. This once again confirms the innate 'knowing' an animal uses when selecting its remedy. It is on this ability that Animal Aromatics is founded. If a medicinal plant is needed, the body will metabolise and utilise it to a great healing effect, if it is not required the body will treat it as a toxin. However, it is still prudent to exercise extra vigilance when using this oil.

Dosage guide
Dogs: initially 1/4 - 1/2 teaspoon per day
Horses: maximum 30ml per day
Cats: inhalation

Carrot
Daucus carota ssp.sativus, D.carota sp.carota

Uses
Liver tonic
Run down animals
Diarrhoea
Older animals especially dogs and horses
Poor hoof / coat conditions

The macerated oil extracted from the root of the common carrot is completely different from carrot seed essential oil which is extracted from the fruit of the wild inedible carrot.

The macerated carrot root oil, rich in beta carotene, is recommended for poor hoof and coat conditions and for animals that are generally run down. Older dogs frequently select it, possibly due to its tonic effects on the liver. Carrot root macerated oil is rich in Vitamins A, B, C, D, E and F and stimulates cell regeneration.

Dosage guide
Dogs and horses: maximum 40 ml per day
Cats: maximum 5 ml per day

> **A cat selects Chickweed**
>
> A cat suffering from a severe skin condition selected chickweed as its only remedy. She drank 10.mls daily for several months, which is excessive for a cat. During this time, her skin completely healed and the steroids she had been given were reduced until she was eventually no longer taking them.

Chickweed
Stellaria media

Uses
Skin disorders, especially in cats
Liver problems / gastrointestinal ulceration
Rheumatic conditions
Protects internal mucus membranes
Bronchitis / congestion

Chickweed is a European plant that is now found as a weed worldwide. It has been used medicinally for centuries. More than 30 species of birds are known to eat both the seeds and the whole plant, hence the common English name 'chick' weed. Chickweed contains triterpene saponins, coumarins, mucilage, gamma-linoleic acid, minerals, flavonoids, organic acids and vitamin C.

The use of chickweed has not been scientifically validated, but it is popular with all animals, especially cats; they tend to select it for a wide variety of problems. The cooling soothing effect that it has on the skin helps relieve itching and other dermal problems and it is not unusual for cats to take large amounts (up to 10 ml in some cases). Chickweed supports the liver and can be selected for rheumatic, lung and stomach problems. Dogs and horses seem partial to both the fresh herb and the macerated oil whereas cats tend to prefer the macerated oil.

Dosage guide
Dogs and horses: maximum 50 ml per day
Cats: maximum 10 ml per day

Chickweed is selected orally or by inhalation to treat the above disorders, it is not applied generally topically.

Comfrey
Symphytum officinale

Uses
Broken bones, fractures, tendons, ligament, cartilage and soft connective tissue damage
Bruising
Arthritis
Inflammation of the stomach and lungs
Coughing

Comfrey is popular with both dogs and horses, particularly those with arthritis. It is a remedy that I would recommend in the tack room or home as it is so useful for sprains, tendon injuries and arthritis.

Comfrey is traditionally known as 'knitbone' because of its ability to aid in the healing of broken bones, fractures, cartilage and soft connective tissue damage. The presence of allantoin is mainly responsible for this action and works by stimulating cell production. Comfrey helps to break down red blood cells, making it a useful remedy for bruising. Its action on the stomach and lungs helps to reduce inflammation and soothe irritation. It is also an expectorant.

Caution: Although comfrey is one of the most widely used plants for healing, there have been concerns about the presence of pyrrolizidine alkaloids found within the plant (the same alkaloids that are found in ragwort and the borage family, of which comfrey is a member). It is believed that over a period of time these alkaloids can have a damaging effect on the liver. However, adverse reactions are only seen when animals are injected with high doses of purified symphytine (the carcinogenic alkaloid found in comfrey) and are not associated with the use of the whole plant. Pyrrolizidine alkaloids are present in higher concentrations in the root than the leaf[12].

Dosage guide
Dogs: maximum 30 ml per day
Horses: maximum 40 ml per day
Cats: maximum 3 ml per day

Linden blossom
Tilia species

Uses
Past abuse
Helps to lift heavy emotions
Anxiety

Linden blossom is an approved herb. It is very popular with dogs, especially those that have suffered abuse. The macerated oil is less potent than the absolute, however, both should be offered to the animal to ascertain which is needed. The effects of linden blossom appear to be sedative and calming, relieving anxiety and restlessness.

Linden flowers contain flavonoids, caffeic (and other acids), mucilage, tannins, volatile oil (0.02-0.1%), traces of benzodiazepine-like compounds, sugar, gum and chlorophyll. A number of flavonoid compounds are also found in linden flowers together with p-coumaric acid. The flavonoids improve circulation.

Dosage guide
Dogs: maximum 40 ml per day
Horses: maximum 40 ml per day
Cats: maximum 5 ml per day

Marigold
Calendula officinalis

Uses
Skin disorders / tissue repair
Stomach / liver disorders
Sadness / comforting

Marigold macerate is very popular with all animals, particularly those with skin and stomach problems relating to depression or anxiety. The marigold belongs to the Asteraceae family the same family as the sunflower. Macerated marigold is anti-spasmodic and is often selected by animals suffering stomach disorders, I have noticed that horses will often select it with devils claw, possibly due to it its protection on the stomach if the properties of devils claw are not needed for its action on the stomach but are for pain. Marigolds are thought to also mimic steroidal effects[6] which possibly attributes to its effectiveness in treating allergy related skin disorders. Amongst other constituents, marigolds also contain saponins; the chemical composition of some saponins is similar to those of human anti-stress and sex hormones from the adrenals and gonads.

The cheerful looking marigold resembling the sun offers feelings of security and comforts a sad heart, lifting depression. In most cases, it is usually taken orally, often in quantities from several licks to 50 ml a time. Topically, calendula also has a reputation for its ability to heal wounds, however, calendula CO_2, extract, which has a dense viscosity is possibly more effective for the treatment of wounds and scar tissue.

Dosage guide
Dogs: maximum 50 ml per day
Horses: maximum 50 ml per day
Cats: maximum 10 ml per day

St John's wort
Hypericum perforatum

Uses
Depression / sedative
Nerve damage
Disorders of the blood, especially viruses
Sarcoids
Liver dysfunction
Vulnerary

St John's wort is a well-known antidepressant and sedative herb. In the Middle Ages, physicians assessed the properties and uses of a plant according to the Doctrine of Signatures. Because the leaves of St John's wort are sprinkled with 'holes' (which resembled wounds), with a colour that look blood-like as the leaf rots, the plant was designated for the treatment of blood conditions. In recent times scientists have established that the red pigment produced by the leaves holds small quantities of a compound called hypericin, which contains an antiviral agent shown to be effective against the HIV virus[13].

St John's wort is very much associated with the blood and viruses transferred by bodily fluids. It arrests bleeding and supports liver function. The macerated oil is a popular remedy with equines. Its photo-toxic properties make it a valuable choice for horses with sarcoids. It is also often selected in cases of nerve damage and inflammation. It is selected by dogs, though less frequently.

Preparations are made from the plant harvested during the flowering season. Constituents include the naphthodianthrones, hypericin and pseudohypericin, flavonoids, xanthones, acylphloroglucinols, volatile oil, procyanidines and caffeic acid derivatives.

Caution:

When offering St John's wort to dogs, check that the dog does not become too drowsy /sedated. If it does, reduce the amount offered to just one eighth of a teaspoon, to produce a relaxed state only.

Do not offer St John's wort if your animal is on any medication, especially sedatives. St. John's wort inhibits the breakdown of serotonin in the body. Do not offer it if there is any type of metabolic problem present in the animal. It is also not recommended for animals prone to photo-sensitivity, however, it may be self-selected by an animal to treat photo-sensitivity (sunburning). Adverse photo-sensitive reactions include blisters, rashes and swollen lips.

It is important to be extra cautious in your observation of dogs selecting St. John's wort.

Dosage guide

Dogs

half a teaspoon twice a day (can be increased to 1 tablespoon in days to follow, provided there is not a deeply sedated reaction).

Horses: maximum 30 ml per day

Cats:: unknown

Fixed oils - the ones used on their own

I do not advise blending essential oils into fixed oils such as flax, hemp and neem as, like the macerated oils, they are a potent remedy in their own right.

Fixed oils	Dog	Cat	Horse
Hemp	very popular	very popular	frequent
Neem	frequent	occasionally	frequent
Flax	very popular	occasionally	frequent

Flax or linseed oil
Linum usitatissimum

Uses

Skin disorders

Colon disorders

Liver problems

Helps prevent cancer

Alleviates the symptoms of arthritis

Gastritis and enteritis

Flax is a blue flowering plant from the Western Canadian Prairies. The fixed oil is extracted from the seeds and is mainly made up of linolenic acid, linoleic acid and oleic acid as well as containing vitamin E and beta carotene (converted to vitamin A by the body), omega-6 and omega-9, essential fatty acids (EFAs), B vitamins, potassium, lecithin, magnesium, fibre, protein and zinc.

Flax seed oil provides approximately 50% more omega-3 fatty acids than fish oil.

Flax seed oil (also known as linseed oil) is frequently selected by dogs with skin and joint disorders and it is sometimes taken in amounts of up to 50 - 70 mls daily. It provides excellent results and is also popular with horses. Most owners will remark on the health and shine of their animals coat when flax oil is selected. Along with spirulina and marigold, it is important to offer flax to animals with skin allergies and joint problems, especially dogs.

EFAs found in the oil are an essential part of the diet as the body is not capable of manufacturing them. They help to relieve arthritis and auto-immune disorders as well as chronic inflammation of the large intestine.

Flax seed oil supports the immune system, circulatory system, reproductive system, nervous system and the joints. It improves liver function which in turn promotes healthy skin, hooves, nails and eyesight. It aids the absorption of calcium and is recommended for constipation. Research shows a low incidence of breast and colon cancer in populations that have high amounts of lignan (such as those found in flaxseeds)[14] in their diet. The oil has been recommended as an aid to eliminating unwanted metals from the body but this is not proven.

Due to the high polyunsaturated fatty acid content of flaxseed oil, this oil is especially prone to rancidity. It should be stored in a cool dark room or in the fridge and used up quickly.

Dosage guide

Dogs and horses: maximum 70 ml per day

Cats: maximum 10 ml per day

Hemp seed oil
Cannabis sativa

Uses

Nervous tension / nerve damage

Dry skin

Hormone imbalance

Arthritis / joint problems

Immune deficiency

Hemp seeds have a history of use for medicine and narcotics and are particulary useful in alleviating skin and joint problems, such as arthritis. Hemp seeds are from the marijuana family but do not contain sufficient quantities of tetrahydrocannabinol (THC) or any other psychoactive substances found in marijuana to make it illegal. Hemp essential oil is also produced and it has similar actions to hemp seed fixed oil.

I would recommend having hemp macerate in stock as it is popular with most animals, especially cats. It supports the nervous system and is often selected for nervous anxiety, offering feelings of peace and tranquillity.

Hemp seeds contain approximately 25% protein, 31% fat (in the form of nutritious oil) and 34% carbohydrates in addition to vitamins and minerals including vitamin E (antioxidant), carotene, phytosterols, calcium, magnesium, sulphur, potassium, phosphorus and trace amounts of iron and zinc. It is also a source of chlorophyll and protein. Hemp mimics enzymes, antibodies, tissues, hormones and blood proteins.

Hemp seed oil also contains 55-70% linoleic acid (LA), 15-25% linolenic acid (LNA) and 10-15% oleic acid. Linoleic and linolenic acids are essential fatty acids (EFAs) that the body is unable to manufacture, so are an important part of the diet. Hemp seed oil contains far greater amounts of antioxidant compounds than flax seed oil. This means that it has a longer shelf-life than flax seed oil, however, flax seed is reported to have much higher concentrations of linolenic acid.

Dosage guide

Dogs and horses: maximum 40 ml per day

Cats: maximum 15 ml per day

A cat with skin problems. Sam Davis

I have used hemp seed with great success on a cat suffering from Malassezia (a yeast infection found in the skin and ears caused by an organism called *Malasezzia pachydermatis*). Just one whiff and the cat went frantic trying to get at the bottle. I think he would have climbed inside, if at all possible! In the past month he has consumed about 500 ml and is still going strong. There has been a significant change in his appearance. His skin, especially on his head, used to be very dry, exfoliating and wrinkled. Now the wrinkles have gone and the skin is looking great. I think the skin was screaming out for all those EFAs.

Neem oil
Azadirachta indica

Uses
Parasites (externally in a gel or shampoo)
Fungal infections (undiluted on isolated areas)
No experience of internal use

The neem tree is native to India. The oil is extracted from the seeds and sold as a cold pressed oil, implying that no heat is used in extraction. However, the extraction process causes a great amount of friction, generating temperatures of around 85°C. Neem oil is bitter to taste and relatively unpalatable.

Neem oil is usually selected by animals infested with or susceptible to parasites. The insect repellent action of neem could be attributed to its insect sterilisation properties. It interferes with the hormone ecdysone and prevents larvae and pupae from completing the molting process[15]. Neem oil therefore provides a hostile environment in which parasites need to multiply, effectively deterring them from the host. As neem does not directly destroy the parasite, future generations of parasites are unlikely to develop resistance to it.

If selected, it is a valuable remedy for conditions such as sweet itch. Neem oil is also thought to stimulate immune responses which in turn helps the body fight against parasites; animals with a compromised immune system will usually be more susceptible. Neem oil has also been found to be deadly to 14 different fungi and has been successful in treating various skin diseases, as well as being capable of treating a wide range of infections including *Staphylococcus*. Nimbin, a constituent of neem oil, was apparently found to be four times as effective as the steroid hydrocortisone[16]. Neem oil could also be useful in a wound gel to deter flies.

Caution: Since neem alters the reproductive function of an insect, apply caution when applying it to breeding and pregnant animals.

Essential Oil Profiles

REVISION

Summary to offering the remedies

Offer aromatics in the recommended order, your animal will then indicate how it wants to proceed. If your animal chooses a number of different oils, offer the ones that work mainly on the mind in the evening and then those that work on the body in the morning.

Offer the aromatics once or twice a day, preferably after feeding. Hold the open bottle firmly in your hand, covering as much of it as possible. When you first offer the remedies, try to introduce the aroma gently, and allow room for your animal to move towards it if they wish. Each animal will react differently, and each will prefer a different intensity of aroma. Watch carefully, and let your animal guide you. Some animals will prefer a space of at least 3 metres between them and the open bottle, while others prefer the bottle to be directly under their nose. Allow your animal to choose how close they wish to be, and to respect their decision.

It is normally safe for chosen remedies to be taken orally. Some animals may turn away from the oils at first, should this occur, you may need to work exclusively with only one or two oils for a few days to open them up to healing. If your animal indicates that it would like to lick the oil, dab a small amount onto your hand and allow it to be licked off. Your animal may wish to self-select by inhalation alone - this is a very potent method of receiving these molecules, as their chemical messages go directly to the brain. Do not try to influence the method of application chosen.

Most animals will want their chosen aromatics for between 3-21 days, but it has been known for them to be taken for much longer. Relax, enjoy, and be observant. Positive signs are different for each animal, and for each issue being dealt with. A slight flaring of a nostril, followed by withdrawal whilst the animal processes the information is a highly positive reaction. Signs of improvement are usually seen within days, and sometimes immediately.

Try to keep records of your animal's interest in the oils. Certain oils contain compounds that may stain fabric or skin – please be cautious. If you have any cause for concern whilst offering aromatics, contact an aromatic professional or vet for advice.

ANGELICA ROOT
Angelica archangelica

Phototoxic, slight dermal irritant
Shelf-life: short / moderate

> **Uses**
> Opens animal to healing
> Sarcoids
> Stomach disturbances / digestive problems
> Stimulates immune function

Most aromatherapy references fail to differentiate between angelica root and angelica seed, giving the impression that the composition is similar, whereas in fact they offer very different therapeutic potential.

The root is selected far more frequently than the seed, possibly because its complex composition offers a larger variety of therapeutic uses. The root contains furanocoumarins which are photo-reactive whereas the seed does not, however, monoterpenes are predominate in both the root and the seed.

Opens animals to healing
Angelica root is popular with all animals especially those that are shut down to healing and not interested in other remedies offered.

Angelica root works deeply within the unconscious mind addressing problems the animal may have experienced during its life, instilling a sense of peace and comfort. As its name suggests, it is the oil of angels, touching deep into the soul.

Sarcoids
Angelica root's photo-reactive properties make it a useful remedy for sarcoids.

Stomach / digestion
Angelica root can help stomach disturbances and digestive problems (caused by spasms). The alcoholic extract is also effective against Listeria[1] (the root only).

APPLICATION AND DILUTIONS. Refer to section on administering the oils

Condition	Topical	Oral	Inhalation	Water Bucket
Opens animal to healing **Stomach disturbances / digestive problems** **Stimulates immune function**		Add 3 -6 drops to 5ml of water	Diluted or undiluted.	Add 3 - 6 drops to water bowl / bucket
Sarcoids	Add approximately 3 - 6 drops to 50ml aloe gel or a clay paste.	as above	as above	as above

BASIL, FRENCH
Ocimum basilicum

Slight oral toxicity, slight dermal irritant
Shelf life: moderate.

> **Uses**
> Physical and mental stimulant
> Stimulates contractions
> Chemically-induced cancer

There are four principal chemotypes of this species of basil but it is the linalol chemotype or French basil, also known as sweet basil that is mainly used in animal therapy.

Contractions
Basil is used to stimulate contractions when the pregnancy has reached full term. Its effects are often rapid and can occur within minutes of inhalation.

Physical and mental stimulant
Basil is also a well-known stimulant of the mind, blood and circulation. It has a warming quality that could be used in muscle rubs, having a dual effect of stimulating blood supply to tired aching muscles.

Scientific research
GST is an enzyme known to be protective against cancer, and 3,4-benzo(a)pyrene is one of the most potent carcinogens in tobacco smoke. Mice were given this chemical to induce cancer and basil was then added to their diet for 14 days. During this time the GST activity significantly increased in the stomach, liver and oesophagus of the mice and the cell carcinoma was significantly reduced. It was concluded that basil essential oil showed considerable promise as a protector against chemically induced cancer[2].

APPLICATION AND DILUTIONS. Refer to section on administering the oils

Condition	Topical	Oral	Inhalation	Water Bucket
Physical and mental stimulant **Chemically induced cancer**		Add 5 -7 drops in 5ml of base oil	Diluted or undiluted.	Add 3 - 5 drops to water bowl / bucket
Stimulates contractions	3-5 drops in 10ml base oil apply in-between back legs where skin is exposed	as above	as above	as above

BAY LAUREL
Laurus nobilis

Non-toxic, slight dermal irritant
Shelf-life: moderate

> **Uses**
> Antiseptic: bacterial and viral infections / mud fever
> Decongestant: lungs / lymphatic system
> Uplifting / self confidence / concentration

Bacteria and viral infections

Bay laurel is popular with horses and is a good antiseptic that has been useful in the treatment of stubborn bacteria and viral infections. Such cases have been seen with mud fever and diseases of the respiratory tract. This effect is possibly due to its complex chemical composition that includes amongst other things, 1,8-cineole and small amounts of phenols.

Decongestant

As bay laurel is produced from the leaves it may account for its affiliation with the lungs since the leaves could be considered the 'lungs' of the tree. Bay laurel is a decongestant which works well on the lymphatic system and swollen lymph nodes.

Behavioural

Bay laurel is uplifting and useful for increasing concentration and confidence.

APPLICATION AND DILUTIONS. Refer to section on administering the oils

Condition	Topical	Oral	Inhalation	Water Bucket
Bacteria and viral infections Decongestant: lungs / lymphatic Uplifting / self confidence	Add 15-20 drops in 150ml watery gel Apply along the windpipe	Add 5-7 drops to 5ml of base oil	Diluted or undiluted	Add 5 - 7 drops to water bowl / bucket
Stimulates contractions	Add to mud fever gel (see recipes)		as above	

BERGAMOT
Citrus bergamia

Non-toxic, photo-reactive
Shelf-life: short / moderate

Uses
Skin disorders: Dry / crusty / flaky
Tumours / sarcoids / growths
Pigment disorders / sun sensitivity
Immune stimulant
Anti-platelet activity
Cardio disorders
Airborne bacteria
Balances body and mind

Bergamot is generally extracted by distillation or cold pressing. It is the cold pressed oils that are normally used in aromatherapy. Even though they contain photo-reactive furanocoumarins such as bergapten, which can result in pigmentation changes and sunburn, they have great therapeutic potential. The distilled bergamot does not contain these photo-reactive compounds because the molecules are too large (heavy) to volatilise.

Avoid applying bergamot in strong sunlight unless it is being used for its photo-reactive properties. Tisserand and Balacs recommend that at least 12 hours should be allowed before the skin can be exposed to sunlight after the application of bergamot[4]. Evenings would therefore be the most appropriate time for its application. The use of bergamot in products that are washed off the coat immediately, such as shampoo, is quite safe and no waiting time for exposure is necessary. If the area where the bergamot has been applied is covered, then exposure to sunlight is not a problem. However, make sure that at least 10 cm in the circumference outside of the application is also covered, due to the migration of the bergamot in the dermal cells.

Greys are more susceptible than other horses to sun burning and they are also more likely to develop tumours for which bergamot will very likely be needed. It is possible to buy bergapten-free bergamot (FCF) but given the choice, the animal will usually select the complete bergamot, which in most cases has a greater therapeutic value. It is perhaps worth stocking both and allowing your animal to choose. Bergamot oil is especially popular with dogs.

Cardio disorders

In an Italian study on the effects of cold pressed *Citrus bergamia* for spasm in the coronary vessels, it was suggested that the furanocoumarins such as bergapten and bergamottin clearly had the potential to be cardio-protective, giving similar results to those of verapamil and other calcium channel-blocking cardiovascular drugs[3].

Dry, flaky, crusty skin / tumours / growths / sarcoids / photo-sensitivity and pigment disorders

Bergamot has a strong association with skin disorders especially when the skin is dry and crusty and has proven invaluable to animals with tumours and sarcoids. In Australia a new photodynamic therapy is being researched, that produces positive results using 'photo-reactive' substances to treat sarcoids[5].

It goes against all logic to even imagine that horses prone to sun burning would select phototoxic oils, but they do. The oils are usually licked in small amounts to alleviate the problem. From my observations, I have formed the opinion that if a plant oil is needed, the body will metabolise and utilise it, rebalancing the affected areas. If it is not required it will throw the body out of balance, causing the symptoms it would otherwise alleviate.

Immune stimulant / airborne bacteria

Research has shown that the major constituents found in bergamot (limonene and related terpenoids) have caused complete regression in the majority of advanced rat mammary cancers when it is added to the diet [6].

Bergamot supports the immune system and is effective against many infectious bacteria. Its volatile nature and anti-bacterial properties gave rise to it once being used extensively in French hospitals to combat infectious airborne bacteria. It should be considered for its effects in preventing the spread of disease in the home, stable yard, whilst travelling or in the waiting room of the veterinary surgery.

A study on bergapten concluded that bergapten had anti-platelet activity [7].

Emotional / behavioural

Bergamot is indicated for moody, irrational behaviour as well as depression and despondency. It uplifts the spirits and disperses repressed emotions that lead to anxiety. Bergamot helps restore physiological and physical balance and uplifts the spirits.

APPLICATION AND DILUTIONS. Refer to section on administering the oils

Condition	Topical	Oral	Inhalation	Water Bucket
Tumours **Sarcoids** **Growths** **Dry/crusty skin** **Pigment disorders** **Sun sensitivity**	Add 10-15 drops to 50ml gel or clay. Apply 1-2 x daily or as needed.	Add 5 -10 drops to 5ml base oil	Diluted or undiluted.	Add 10 -20 drops to a water bucket
Balancing Mental & Physical body		as above	as above	
Immune Stimulant		as above	as above	
Airborne Bacteria				Add 15-30 drops to 150ml water. Use as a spray or add 10-20 drops to a water bucket

CARROT SEED, WILD
Daucus carota

Non-toxic, slight dermal irritant
Shelf Life: Moderate

> **Uses**
> Internal bleeding
> Wounds that are slow to heal
> Cell damage
> Liver damage or malfunction
> Coat and hoof conditioner
> Poor appetite / malnutrition
> Immune stimulant
> Tumours: sarcoids / cysts

Wild carrot, or Queen Anne's lace, is a small inedible wild carrot that has a tough whitish root, quite different from the cultivated *Daucus carota* var. *sativa,* that gives us the edible root. The essential oil is extracted by distillation from the fruits of wild carrot and the macerated oil is obtained by the root of the common edible cultivated carrot being left to soak in a vegetable oil, which contains high concentrations of carotenes. Do not confuse carrot macerated root with carrot seed essential oil, as they offer very different properties.

Carrot seed essential oil is popular with horses, which perhaps ties in with their association to the carrot. Its acrid taste does not reflect its earthy aroma, yet the animal will repeatedly lick the oil until the required amount has been taken; horses will often take relatively large doses of this oil in comparison to other essential oils. Dogs and cats respond less frequently to carrot seed but will select it when needed.

Internal bleeding / Wounds that are slow to heal / Cell damage

Carrot seed appears to stimulate platelet activity and has proven to be invaluable where there is internal bleeding such as pulmonary haemorrhaging and also for internal cell damage caused by rattle snake bites, an operation or other similar complications. Carrot seed assists the body in repairing itself, possibly by its effect on the liver, by stimulating healthy cells, thereby aiding the animal's recovery. Wounds that are slow to heal also respond well to carrot seed both as an oral or topical remedy, however, external applications for cell repair usually require lavender oil.

Liver damage or malfunction

Animals will normally select carrot seed when the liver is not functioning efficiently. Its application for disorders of the liver is well known, and research has shown that carotol, the main constituent of carrot seed, is responsible for stimulating the regeneration of liver cells, which in turn aids in the detoxification of the blood.

Coat and hoof conditioner

Where there are skin problems or a yellowish discolouration to the nails, it is prudent to check the health of the liver. Toxins due to liver malfunction could result in their being excreted through the dermal layers, causing irritation, whether taken orally or inhaled. The effects that carrot seed has had in repairing damaged, dry and cracked hoofs, have been dramatic.

A five-year old horse that was born with a cloven hoof needed to have it stapled together with six staples. However after two weeks of applying a macerated base oil with carrot seed essential oil daily to the hoof, it bound together. The farrier no longer needed to use staples as there was only about one inch left of the cloven hoof. The horse was also inhaling carrot seed and seaweed throughout the treatment.

Immune stimulant / Tumours / Sarcoids / Poor appetite / Malnutrition

Carrot seed is a valuable oil for animals that are run down and for those that have lost condition. Starvation or diseases that have caused weight loss, or malnutrition both past and present, as well as loss of appetite, will all indicate carrot seed. It is a good immune stimulant and is often needed orally where there are tumours, cysts or sarcoids.

Note

Carrot seed is an essential oil that may be needed in a stronger application, in some cases when a 50% dilution appears too weak (indicated by taking a 5ml dose and still looking for more) the horse will benefit from the oil being offered undiluted in its natural state.

APPLICATION AND DILUTIONS. Refer to section on administering the oils

Condition	Topical	Oral	Inhalation	Water Bucket
Coat & hoof Conditioner	Add 10-20 drops to 50 ml of base oil, preferably macerated carrot. Apply 1-2 x daily to the hoof or as needed	Add 10-30 drops to 5 ml of base oil. In cases where the animal wants the whole bottle, make a 50% dilution	Diluted or undiluted.	Add 20- 30 drops to a water bucket
Tumours: Sarcoids, cysts		as above	as above	as above
Internal bleeding Wounds slow to heal/cell damage Poor appetite Immune disorders Liver damage		as above	as above	

CHAMOMILE, GERMAN
Matricaria recutita

Non-toxic:, non-irritant
Shelf Life: moderate

Uses
- Allergies - histamine
- Inflamed conditions (internal & external)
- Skin eruptions
- Respiratory disorders (inflammation)
- Anxiety / tension

Antihistaminic / anti-inflammatory
German chamomile contains alpha-bisabolol, a sesquiterpene alcohol, and also chamazulene, which characterises its ink-blue colour. Both of these constituents are responsible for the oil's strong anti-inflammatory and antihistamine properties. German chamomile is quite different in its composition and effect to Roman chamomile which contains comparatively small amounts of azulene and no alpha-bisabolol. Approximately 50% of German chamomile is made up of alpha-bisabolol which has an even stronger anti-inflammatory effect than azulene.

Skin eruptions and stomach disorders usually of a nervous, anxious origin
German chamomile is indicated for conditions where the skin is inflamed, raw or broken and where an anti-inflammatory or antihistamine action is needed and also for insect bites. Yarrow which works in a similar anti-inflammatory way but generally on wounds (and for emotional release) may also help such conditions. Offer both oils to the animal to ascertain which will be the more effective as they may both be needed. German chamomile is generally selected where the name of the condition ends in 'itis', such as colitis, laminitis. German chamomile also encourages granulation and tissue regeneration, providing very beneficial results in the treatment of proud flesh.

German chamomile is commonly selected for disorders of the stomach, especially where there is inflammation of a nervous origin.

Immune response
Ingestion of either Roman or German chamomile is thought to stimulate the production of white blood corpuscles (leucocytes) that help fight infection.

Respiratory disorders of a nervous, anxious origin
Respiratory distress caused by allergens very often benefits from German chamomile, which offers both antihistaminic and anti-inflammatory properties. If the condition is severe, the animal will most likely choose great mugwort, then as the symptoms begin to improve, change over to German chamomile. Great mugwort and German chamomile contain sesquiterpenes.

Scientific research
Azulene, a constituent of German chamomile, has noted bacteriostatic properties. At a strength of 1 part to 2000, it is effective against *Staphylococcus aureus* and haemolytic streptococcus (an agent of scarlet fever and acute rheumatoid arthritis). Infected wounds

have been healed using a concentration of 1 - 85,000 [8].

A report from Tokyo showed that by inhaling German chamomile essential oil, *Matricaria chamomilla,* there was significant reduction in the levels of plasma ACTH in stressed rats. ACTH (adrenocorticotrophic hormone), is released from the anterior pituitary gland in response to stress. When the benzodiazepine receptors were blocked, there was no effect from the chamomile oil inhalation. This conclusively demonstrates that chamomile is acting via benzodiazepine-sensitive receptors [9].

APPLICATION AND DILUTIONS. Refer to section on administering the oils

Condition	Topical	Oral	Inhalation	Water Bucket
Skin: **Raw** **Eruptions** **Inflamed** **Allergies** **Proud flesh** **Staphylococcus aureus**	Apply undiluted or add 10 - 15 drops to 50 ml gel	Add 4 -8 drops to 5ml of base oil	Diluted or undiluted.	
Respiratory: **Allergy** **Anxiety** **Streptococcus**	Add 10-15 drops to 150ml gel, apply to neck, dab on nostrils. Use diluted or undiluted.	as above	as above	
Stomach: **Inflammation** **Anxiety**	Add 5 - 10 drops to 50ml gel. Apply to belly area in between the back legs.	as above	as above	
Immune Response		as above	as above	

CHAMOMILE, ROMAN
Anthemis nobilis / Chamaemelum nobile

Non-toxic, non-irritant
Shelf life: Moderate

> **Uses**
> Anxious - nervous temperament
> Skin disorders of an anxious origin
> Stomach disorders - anxiety related

Anxious / nervous temperament.
When an animal with a history of skin problems or stomach disorders displays an anxious temperament, they usually select Roman chamomile. Tense, hard muscles are also an indication that Roman chamomile may be needed. It is a soothing, relaxing oil with a pronounced effect on the nervous system, aiding sleep and relaxation.

Skin disorders: Nervous, anxious origin
Roman chamomile is frequently used for skin disorders linked to anxiety. There is often confusion over the specific uses of the two chamomiles regarding skin problems. German chamomile is generally applied to the inflamed damaged skin and is characterised by its ink-blue colour. It has stronger anti-inflammatory and antihistaminic properties than the pale green Roman chamomile that is used to treat the root emotional cause for the presenting skin disorder. This is usually inhaled or taken orally, which is generally more effective than topical application. Its action is thought to be achieved by activating messages to the brain's limbic (emotional) centre.

Stomach disorders: Anxiety
Roman chamomile is mainly composed of esters, which calm the nervous system and give it its powerful antispasmodic effect. It can therefore be very beneficial to stress-related conditions of the digestive tract such as spasmodic colic and loose droppings.

APPLICATION AND DILUTIONS Roman Chamomile Refer to section on administering the oils

Condition	Topical	Oral	Inhalation	Water Bucket
Skin: **Related to nervous anxiety** **Dry Irritated & angry**	Add 5-10 drops to 50ml gel, or add to a natural shampoo Caution: Water and oil can aggravate certain skin conditions	Add 5-10 drops to 5ml of base oil or water Note: Bald patches normally respond better when treated orally or by inhalation	Diluted or undiluted.	Add 5-10 drops in a bucket of water
Stomach Nervous anxiety		Add 5-10 drops to 5ml of base oil or water	as for above	as for above
Anxiety	Dab onto paws, poll / forehead, chest or nostrils undiluted or diluted	as for above	as for above	as for above

CLARY SAGE
Salvia sclarea

Non-toxic, non-irritant
Shelf life: moderate

> **Uses**
> Hormone balancing (possibly contains phyto hormones)
> Birthing
> Nervous anxiety

Do not confuse clary sage with common or garden sage *Salvia officinalis* which has a high ketone (thujone) content. Clary sage is generally selected by nervous animals, the type that would perhaps also select violet leaf. However, even though violet leaf is more popular, clary sage seems to be selected when nervous, behaviour and mood swings are associated with a hormone imbalance.

Salvatore Battaglia explains 'The oil is one of several that promotes oestrogen secretion and is believed to act on the pituitary. Its analgesic effects and ability to accelerate labour may make it useful in giving birth'[10].

Clary sage is a deeply relaxing oil and is also suited to over excitable or stressed animals, calming the mind and easing tension.

APPLICATION AND DILUTIONS. Refer to section on administering the oils

Condition	Topical	Oral	Inhalation	Water Bucket
Hormone regulator Nervous anxiety		Add 5-7 drops to 5ml base oil	Diluted or undiluted.	Add 3-6 drops to water bowl / bucket
During labour	3-5 drops in 10ml base oil apply in-between back legs where skin is exposed	as above	as above	

EUCALYPTUS
Eucalyptus radiata

Generally non-toxic, non-irritant
Shelf-life: moderate

> **Uses**
> Winter chills / fever / respiratory
> Insecticide: helps to deter insects
> Bacteria / viruses

There are over seven hundred species of eucalyptus recorded. The many species of gum tree, as they are known, dominate the Australian flora. *Eucalyptus globulus* is the species most commonly used in aromatherapy, producing an essential oil with good all round effects. However *Eucalyptus radiata* produces a finer smelling essential oil that is rich in 1,8-cineole.

Eucalyptus is not an oil that is frequently selected by horses and it is less frequently selected by dogs and cats, however it should not be overlooked in its value for respiratory conditions and fever.

Respiratory / fever

The principal use of *Eucalyptus radiata* is to treat respiratory problems, especially those associated with fever, due to its cooling effect on the body. Its expectorant activity may be directly linked to the 1,8-cineole content, which provides properties that loosen mucus and reduce swelling of the mucus membranes, making breathing easier. *Eucalyptus radiata* can also be used to treat asthmatic conditions, but be careful to make sure that the animal has a strong attraction to its aroma. An unwanted application can trigger an attack, producing the symptoms that it would otherwise help.

Bactericide / antiviral

For thousands of years the Aboriginal Australians had knowledge of the medicinal uses of the leaves of the eucalyptus tree. They knew that there would be no or little infection if they were to bind eucalyptus leaves round even serious wounds and that healing would be rapid. Kurt Schnaubelt writes [11] that the 3-4% of aldehydes present in eucalyptus radiata lend an especially broad spectrum of action (antiviral, expectorant, anti-inflammatory). Tisserand states that, a 2% emulsion of eucalyptus sprayed into a room will kill 70% of airborne staphylococci [12].

Insecticide

Eucalyptus trees are often found in areas where there is a density of mosquitoes, for which they provide the antidote. The tree emits a substance that deters mosquitoes and the essential oil is effective against malaria.

Even though eucalyptus oil generally deters insects, it is not a sure indication that it should be applied to your animal. Indeed many animals have an adverse reaction to its application. One dog was seen to be crying running in circles after the application of this oil so - as with all oils - ask your animal first.

APPLICATION AND DILUTIONS. Refer to section on administering the oils

Condition	Topical	Oral	Inhalation	Water Bucket
Respiratory fever	Add 8-10 drops to 150ml of loose gel. Apply to the windpipe / chest **Caution**: Asthma	Add 5-10 drops to 5ml of base oil or water	Diluted or undiluted.	Add 3-5 drops in a bowl or 7-10 drops in a bucket of water
Bacterial /viral infections	Add 5-10 drops to 50ml of gel or water. Apply as needed	as above	as above	as above
Insecticide	Use aromatic eucalyptus water or add 15-20 drops to 150ml of water. Use as a spray or wipe on the coat. Apply as needed		as above	

FENNEL
Foeniculum vulgare var. *amara*
Foeniculum vulgare var. *dulce*

Slightly-toxic, slight dermal irritant

Shelf-life: moderate

> **Uses**
> Colic
> Digestive problems
> Balances female hormones
> Lactation

Two varieties of fennel are used in animal therapy, common or bitter fennel, which is found in wild or cultivated states and sweet fennel, which is always cultivated. These should not be confused with a third type of fennel which is known as Florence fennel *Foeniculum azoricum*. Both the common and bitter fennel have their place in therapy. The bitter fennel is more potent and appears to be frequently needed, but extra caution needs to be maintained when using it, due to its fenchone content.

Balances female hormones
Fennel has an influential effect on oestrogen activity, which is possibly due to the oil's anethole content. It seems to have the ability to balance lactation by encouraging or discouraging milk supply.

Digestive problems
Fennel has been used through the centuries as an appetite suppressant and diuretic. It is an effective antispasmodic of the gastric and intestinal smooth muscle, stimulating and calming the digestive tract, depending on what is needed. This makes it a useful remedy for animals prone to spasmodic colic and indeed it is used in many pharmaceutical preparations for such disorders.

Caution: Topical over use of fennel can cause skin irritation and sensitisation. This is exacerbated in water.

APPLICATION AND DILUTIONS. Refer to section on administering the oils

Condition	Topical	Oral	Inhalation	Water Bucket
Colic **Digestion** **Female hormones** **Lactation**		Add 5-7 drops to 5ml base oil	Diluted or undiluted.	Add 3-6 drops to water bowl / bucket

FLOUVE, ABSOLUTE
Anthoxanthum odoratum

Non-toxic, non-irritant
Shelf life: moderate

Uses
Sedative
Allergies
Immune stimulant

Flouve is produced from fresh grasses. It seems to work via the principle of 'like cures like' and has been successful in the treatment of allergies caused by hay, grasses and pollens. These allergens very often affect the respiratory tract and skin and can also cause problems such as headshaking.

Flouve contains high levels of coumarins, which in excess can cause liver damage, but in moderation coumarins are used for the treatment of lymphoedema and various cancers. They are reported to be immune stimulants with anti-platelet activity (blood thinning).[13] Various coumarins have antiphlogistic and circulatory stimulant properties, and others are spasmolytic or sedative. They can also have antibacterial properties.

APPLICATION AND DILUTIONS. Refer to section on administering the oils

Condition	Topical	Oral	Inhalation	Water Bucket
Sedative **Allergies** **Immuno stimulant**		Add 5-7 drops to 5ml base oil	Diluted or undiluted.	Add 3-6 drops to water bowl / bucket

FRANKINCENSE
Boswellia carterii

Non-toxic, non-irritant
Shelf life: moderate

> **Uses**
> Lungs
> Intestinal problems of
> an emotional origin (diarrhoea)
> Fear

Frankincense has been used since ancient times in religious ceremonies and is mentioned in the Bible 22 times. The word 'franc' comes from 'pure' or 'free' and 'incensium' from 'smoke'. It has been discovered that when frankincense is burned it produces a mind altering substance (which expands the sub-consciousness).

There are many grades of frankincense. The finest quality is produced from the carefully selected 'tears' while the ungraded oil is taken from the bark, dust and siftings.

Behavioural: fear / intestinal problems of an emotional origin

Frankincense helps to distance the animal from fear, helping it to calm and centre itself by taking the mind away from commotion into a more peaceful place. Frankincense is indicated when the animal is genuinely frightened rather than highly strung. The fear may be related to something that happened in the past as well as the present situation. As with sandalwood, rose and angelica, frankincense will also help the animal pass into the next world at the time of death.

Frankincense is excellent for the treatment of fear and anxiety-related diarrhoea.

Lung problems

Frankincense encourages long, slow, deep breathing, which in itself is a well known calming technique. It possesses anti-catarrhal and expectorant properties making it useful against bronchitis and asthma.

APPLICATION AND DILUTIONS. Refer to section on administering the oils

Condition	Topical	Oral	Inhalation	Water Bucket
Lungs **Related to grief anxiety**	Dab diluted or undiluted onto poll / forehead, paws or nostrils	Add 5-10 drops to 5ml base oil or water	Diluted or undiluted	Add 10 - 15 drops in a bucket / bowl of water
Behavioural / fear **Large intestine**	as above	as above	as above	as above

GARLIC
Allium sativum

Generally non-toxic, dermal irritant
Shelf life : moderate / long

Uses
Airborne bacteria
Respiratory disorders
Parasites / sweet itch / mud fever
Fly repellent
Immune stimulant
Antibacterial
Abscesses
Dilates blood capillaries
Blood thinning
Circulation / arthritis / navicular / ringbone
Laminitis

Garlic is favoured by horses more than by dogs and cats.

Airborne bacteria
The vapour of garlic essential oil provides a hostile environment for bacteria and it has long been recognised for its effect in warding off infection. Sprayed into the air, it can be a potent precautionary measure to guard against airborne bacteria, which is especially useful when animals have been in contact with infected animals.

Respiratory disorders
Most essential oils are excreted through the faeces, urine, skin and lungs. However, garlic is primarily evacuated through the lungs. Its strong antiseptic properties offer a powerful remedy in cases of severe lung infection and its use is indicated for acute and chronic respiratory problems. These include COPD, infection, equine flu, bronchitis, lung worm, a persistent cough and pneumonia. I have found that almost all COPD cases respond to garlic. Garlic essential oil is chemically quite different from the garlic flakes or powders. This would explain why it is not uncommon for animals such as horses to be partial to the garlic essential oil, even when they have shown no or little interest in garlic flakes and powders.

Parasites: sweet itch / mud fever
Externally, garlic repels mites and midges and helps prevent reinfestation. Its use is especially indicated in cases of sweet itch to deter mites, help ease the itch and to help prevent secondary infection. Garlic is also effective against the *Dermatophilus congolensis* bacterium that cause conditions such as mud fever and rain scald[14]. Garlic should normally be used in conjunction with either yarrow or German chamomile to counteract its harsh effect on the skin.

A study by Alisha Yardley on *D. congolensis* showed that one tenth of a drop of garlic caused complete bacterial elimination. While thyme, lavender and povidone iodine (commercial product) had some effect, they were not able to totally inhibit the bacteria (refer to chart in this section).[14]

Immune system / antibacterial
A Bangladeshi team studied garlic extract and allicin, a constituent of it, against four of the most significant enterotoxic bacteria which cause dysentery and cholera including *Shigella*

dysenteriae, S.flexneri, enterotoxigenic Escherichia coli and *Vibrio cholerae*.[15] Both the allicin and the garlic extract were highly active in vitro against all 40 strains of the four bacteria species tested. The conventional drugs Ampicillin, Co-trimoxazole and Tetracycline, were mostly useless against the bacteria. Only Gentamycin (which is very toxic to the kidneys and the auditory system) had the same range of activity as the garlic preparations.

Garlic has long been used for its effectiveness in fighting infection, particularly of the respiratory tract, but also of the blood and other tissues. Other recent evidence has found that garlic enhances the immune system by its effect on white blood cells and T-helper cells, which promote antigen-specific immune responses, and NK cells that are important in non-specific immune responses and in neutralising anti-cancer cells[16]. The essential oil appeared more powerful than garlic powder or flakes.

Another research team compared the antibacterial activity of allicin and aqueous garlic extracts with the antibiotics ampicillin and kanamycin[17]. Results showed that garlic treatments were as effective as the antibiotics. Allicin and garlic extract showed activity against 19 out of 20 strains of Gram-positive and Gram-negative organisms.

The complex nature of an essential oil would make it hard for bacteria to develop simultaneous resistance to more than one of its active ingredients, as opposed to the synthetic structure of an antibiotic. Garlic is a very potent remedy for abscesses and puncture wounds, particularly in the foot.

Dilates blood capillaries / aids circulation / arthritis / navicular / ringbone / laminitis

Garlic helps to clean the blood and dilates the capillaries. Its anti-platelet (blood thinning) activity makes it useful in treating navicular and similar conditions where the circulation has been severely reduced.

Caution

Garlic inhibits iodine metabolism and blood clotting. Avoid using with animals awaiting surgery; it increases the chance of haemorrhage.

Undiluted garlic is very irritating to the skin and mucus membranes. Always dilute into a fixed oil if it is being taken by mouth, or a gel with anti-inflammatory oils such a yarrow or German chamomile if applied topically.

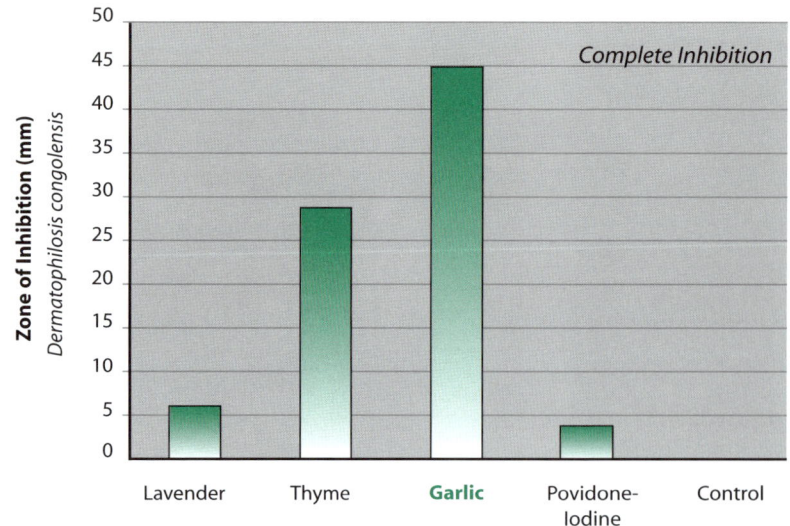

All compounds, with exception to the controls, produced a zone of inhibition of growth of dermatophilosis congolensis due to the application of essential oils or povidone-iodine. Garlic exerted the most inhibitory effects, showing complete inhibition of growth, followed by thyme, lavender and povidone-iodine in that order. There was no inhibition of growth from distilled water (controls) indeed growth was even and profuse.

Extract from a 2001 project by Alisha Yardley, subsequently published in the International Journal of Aromatherapy (2004).[14]

APPLICATION AND DILUTIONS. Refer to section on administering the oils

Condition	Topical	Oral	Inhalation	Water Bucket
Skin: **Sweet Itch** **Mud fever** **Parasites**	Add 10-15 drops to 150ml gel, add equal quantities of an azulene oil (blue). Plus other needed oils. Apply to the affected area 1-2 x daily or as needed	Add 5-8 drops to 5ml of base oil	Diluted or undiluted	
Respiratory disorders **Airborne bacteria**		as above	Add 8-10 drops to 150ml water. Use as a spray	Add 10 drops to a bucket of water. Mix well. Use mainly for farm animals
Dilates the blood capillaries **Aids circulation**		as above	Diluted or undiluted	
Immune system		as above	as above	as above
Abscesses **Puncture wounds**	Apply undiluted, to the foot only, directly onto the affected area. Apply 2-3 x daily or as needed	as above	as above	

GERANIUM
Pelargonium graveolens

Non-toxic, non-irritant

Shelf life: moderate

> **Uses**
> Balancing to mind and body
> Balances hormones (thought to contain phyto hormones)
> Relieves congestion

Geranium, like bergamot, is balancing to both the mind and body. It has a stimulating effect on the adrenals and a regulating effect on the hormones. While bergamot is masculine, geranium is feminine.

Geranium is relatively popular with animals. One horse I worked with took a few sniffs of geranium and no sooner had I turned my back than she was laid out flat on the ground in her stable. Thankfully, the owner reassured me that her horse did this when very relaxed!

Geranium has a balancing effect on the nervous system and relieves anxiety and depression. It also relieves congestion and is haemostatic which means it helps to arrest bleeding.

APPLICATION AND DILUTIONS. Refer to section on administering the oils

Condition	Topical	Oral	Inhalation	Water Bucket
Balancing / mind and body **Regulates hormones** **Relieves congestion** **Behavioural / fear** **Large intestine**		Add 5-7 drops to 5ml base oil or water	Diluted or undiluted	Add 3-6 drops to water bowl / bucket

IMMORTELLE
Helichrysum angustifolium

Non-toxic, non-irritant
Shelf life: moderate / long

Uses
- Emotionally deprived
- Cellular growth / proud flesh / scar tissue
- Bruises - disperses old blood
- Diuretic
- Mucus conditions

Immortelle, also known as everlasting or helichrysum, thrives well in hot sunny climates.

It offers feelings of warmth and love from the sun's rays and is suited to animals that have lacked love and attention as well as those that lack confidence.

Immortelle helps to loosen adhesions from wounds and scars and is excellent for stimulating cellular growth. Topically, it promotes the healing of bruises and scar tissue, and it is also effective for the treatment of proud flesh.

Immortelle has a stimulating effect on the spleen, liver, gall bladder and kidneys; the organs that are responsible for cleaning the body. In traditional aromatherapy, helichrysum essential oil is often used for liver disorders.

Immortelle has an antibacterial action. It also contains sesquiterpenes that are anti-inflammatory and small chain ketones that might offer mucolytic properties.

APPLICATION AND DILUTIONS. Refer to section on administering the oils

Condition	Topical	Oral	Inhalation	Water Bucket
Emotional **Diuretic**		Add 3-5 drops to 5ml base oil	Diluted or undiluted.	
Mucus conditions	5 -10 drops in 150ml watery gel (with other needed oils) applied to the windpipe	as above	as above	
Cellular growth **Proud flesh** **Scar tissue** **Bruises**	5 -7 drops in 50ml firm gel applied to the area			

JASMINE ABSOLUTE
Jasminum grandiflorum

Non-toxic, generally non-irritant
Shelf life: long

Uses
Deeply calming / comforting
Vices
Tense and nervous behaviour
Deprived of affection / neglect
Male dominant behaviour
Male / female reproductive balance

In India, jasmine is known as the Queen of the Night, as her flowers are hand-picked after dusk and before dawn, when their fragrance is most potent. Virtually all jasmine oil is produced as an absolute or CO_2 extraction rather than as an essential oil. For every kilo of oil produced, 1000 kilos of hand picked blossoms are required, for this reason it is not possible to buy an inexpensive bottle of jasmine absolute. As with other precious oils, if it is too cheap it has most probably been adulterated.

Vices and tense behaviour

Jasmine takes on the heightened emotions of the night, embracing sensuality. It comforts fears and instills a sense of calm, innocence and peace. The deeply relaxing and comforting qualities of jasmine make it a useful remedy for calming the mind, body and spirit.

Captive animals very often develop vices in an attempt to release endorphins to help ease the frustration of confinement. In such cases, jasmine may be useful. It helps to alleviate feelings of nervous anxiety and boredom that can result from restraint, offering feelings of security and warmth, thus easing vices. Jasmine should also be offered where there may have been neglect or where there is restless depression. It puts the mind in touch with its deepest self, helping to re-establish trust.

Reproductive problems

Jasmine balances male energy as rose balances female energy, although is frequently selected by females during birth and lactation. Jasmine appears to encourage sexual activity, which is possibly due to its effect in lessening anxiety and its ability to influence and balance hormonal activity. The effect jasmine can have on contractions make it a useful remedy during prolonged labour and it can also help with the bonding of mother and off-spring. Such actions would suggest that breeders may benefit from keeping jasmine stock.

Male dominant behaviour

Jasmine is also effective in treating aggressive, dominant 'bully' behaviour, which may be associated with insecurity or hormone imbalance.

APPLICATION AND DILUTIONS. Refer to section on administering the oils

Condition	Topical	Oral	Inhalation	Water Bucket
Colic **Digestion** **Female hormones** **Lactation**		Add 5-7 drops to 5ml base oil	Diluted or undiluted.	Add 3-6 drops to water bowl / bucket

JUNIPER BERRY
Juniperus communis

Non-toxic, non-irritant
Shelf life: moderate

Uses
Urinary / kidney
Fluid retention
Blood - detoxifying / anti-microbial
Helps rid lactic and uric acid from the body
Arthritis / stressed muscles
Mental stagnation
Lack of self worth
Emotional neglect
Trying to please

Juniper berry essential oil is superior to juniper essential oil as it is extracted from the berries only, whilst juniper essential oil can be extracted from the whole plant, usually this means the leaves and twigs. Juniper grows in very varied conditions such as moorlands, mountains and coniferous forests.

Its antiseptic properties have been known since prehistoric times and it is believed to be one of the earliest medicines used by man. The Romans used juniper for controlling contagious diseases and for disinfecting the air, and our forefathers used to grind up the berries and add them to the feed of their horses, as it was thought to 'ginger them up'. Early records of juniper are mentioned in Black's Veterinary Dictionary published in 1928; under the heading Gin (which is juniper-based) it quotes its use as a 'diuretic in cases where the urine is scanty'.[20]

Urinary / kidney / antimicrobial activity
Juniper is one of the most useful oils for kidney and bladder problems. These can be characterised by excessive thirst and urination, horses may display uncharacteristic bucking when ridden. Juniper is a detoxifying remedy and one of its main functions is to support the kidneys, which in turn filter waste from the body. It is especially indicated for urinary problems that are possibly caused by toxins.

A study on the antimicrobial activity of different juniper oils showed that alpha-terpineol was its strongest most active constituent, found in good amounts in various species (such as Juniperus oxycedrus). It was active against *Bacillus cereus* and very active against *B. subtilis*, *Escherichia coli*, *Micrococcus luteus*, *Staphylococcus aureus*, *Staphylococcus epidermidis* and *Candida albicans*[21]. Another study revealed that juniper is traditionally used for its diuretic properties as it is believed to enhance glomerular filtration[22].

Fluid retention / arthritis / stressed muscles
Juniper berry is one of the most useful oils for fluid retention, a condition frequently seen in horses' legs after periods of box rest. It is a valuable oil for arthritic conditions and stressed aching muscles.

Juniper berry inhibits cold and damp from penetrating into the body while also helping to clear excess uric and lactic acid from the system. Arthritic conditions may also benefit from a topical application with the addition of oils such as birch, wintergreen or peppermint in a gel base, to ease the pain. Yarrow can also be added for its anti-inflammatory properties.

Celery seed essential oil, which has a similar application and use to juniper berry, is sometimes selected orally by horses for arthritic conditions.

Misconceptions about juniper oil

Juniper berries *(Juniperus communis)* and the essential oil derived from them, have long been indicated as a useful diuretic, supporting kidney function. However, juniper and other high-terpene hydrocarbon containing essential oils have been suggested as being kidney irritants. It appears that the origin of such statements, which are still mentioned in a number of aromatherapy texts, came from large, fatal doses of juniper oil given to dogs. These high doses caused clouding of the urine, which was then assumed to be due to kidney damage. However, it appears that the cloudiness was due to the presence of large quantities of juniper oil metabolites[23]. More recent studies including those on laboratory rats have found no kidney damage, even when high doses of juniper oil were given[24].

Juniper essential oil also appears to have been confused with Savin (*Juniperus Sabina*) due to the similarity of the Latin names. Savin is an abortifacient.

APPLICATION AND DILUTIONS. Refer to section on administering the oils

Condition	Topical	Oral	Inhalation	Water Bucket
Urinary / Kidney		Add 5-10 drops to 5ml of fixed oil or water	Diluted or undiluted	Add 5-10 drops to a bucket or bowl of water
Fluid filled legs Arthritis Stressed muscles	Add 15-25 drops to 150ml loose watery gel Apply 1-2 x daily or as needed	as above	as above	as above
Blood purifier Latic & uric acid Toxins		as above	as above	as above
Behavioural		as above	as above	as above

LAVENDER
*Lavandula officinalis /
Lavandula angustifolia*

Non-toxic, non-irritant
Shelf life: moderate

Uses
Comforting
Wounds / scars / proud flesh
Insect bites
Respiratory
Birthing / reproductive
Muscular aches
Irritability
Obsessive worry
Nervous anxiety
Withdrawal

The name *Lavandula* comes from the Latin word lavare, which means 'to wash', indicating an association with cleansing and disinfecting. The Greeks and the Romans used it to disinfect wounds, sick rooms and hospital wards. The various species of lavender used by the therapist are listed below.

True lavender (wild or cultivated) comes from *L. officinalis* (synonymous with *L. angustifolia*). True lavender is typically a mountain plant and is characterised by its rich composition in alcohols such as linalol and esters such as linalyl acetate. This is an essential oil with confirmed sedative and analgesic properties.

Spike lavender comes from *Lavandula latifolia* (synonymous with *L. spica*). This is a species that grows at lower altitudes and has a typically camphoraceous scent owing to the presence of camphor and 1,8-cineole. It has remarkable analgesic properties and has been included in veterinary preparations for a number of years such as for infestation, wounds and arthritic complaints.

Lavandin is *Lavandula x intermedia* and is a naturally occurring hybrid of true lavender and spike lavender. It is now cultivated on a large scale. It is extremely versatile as it has a rich composition that reflects both true and spike lavenders.

Behavioural
True lavender can offer comfort and calm to an animal; it is gently yet deeply relaxing and is associated with symptoms of withdrawal. It can also help to break habits and has been effective in easing irritability by releasing pent up energy. Lavender is also selected by over sensitive animals.

Proud flesh
Lavender stimulates the regeneration of skin tissues. It has antioxidant properties that help to prevent scarring and proud flesh. The analgesic properties of lavender offer added benefit, as does its ability to disinfect wounds. Application is usually undiluted or applied in an aloe vera gel, which in itself can enhance the treatment.

Insect bites, mites, flies
Lavender can work well as an insect repellent and remedy for insect bites and is generally non-offensive to most animals.

Respiratory

Emotional disturbances manifested in the lungs can benefit from *Lavandula officinalis*. According to Tisserand[25], vapourised lavender will destroy *Pneumococcus* and haemolytic *Streptococcus* within 12 - 24 hours, and it is also recommended for conditions such as asthma and bronchitis. Spike lavender is a good choice for its expectorant effect, dissolving sputum. It can reduce pain and swelling and improve blood sedimentation and mobility.

Reproductive / foaling

There are instances where lavender has been used to help animals with a history of miscarriages. It must be stressed, however, that any expectant animal must make a positive move toward the oil. Lavender can also help with tearing during the birth, while also having a relaxing effect on the mother and the new born.

Muscular aches

Lavender's antispasmodic, relaxant and analgesic properties make it a useful remedy for the treatment of tired, aching or sore muscles.

APPLICATION AND DILUTIONS. Refer to section on administering the oils

Condition	Topical	Oral	Inhalation	Water Bucket
Wounds **Ringworm** **Scars** **Proud flesh** **Insect bites**	Apply undiluted Ringworm use undiluted or add 10-20 drops to 50ml of gel	Add 5-8 drops to 5ml of base oil	Diluted or undiluted	
Behavioural	Apply undiluted or diluted to the poll / forehead, chest or nostrils	as above	Add 8-10 drops to 150ml water. Use as a spray	Add 10 drops to a bucket of water. Mix well. Use mainly for farm animals
Reproductive Foaling / tearing	Apply to the tear undiluted or dilute 10-20 drops into 50ml aloe vera gel. It can also be applied using a spray	as above	Diluted or undiluted	as above
Tired muscles	Add 20-30 drops to 150ml gel. Apply 1-2 x daily or as needed			

LEMON
Citrus limon

Non-toxic, slight dermal irritant
Shelf life: short

Uses
Uplifting /aids concentration
Kidney stones
Uric and lactic acid
Immuno-stimulant
Balances hormones
Cleansing

Lemon is an inexpensive oil with a multitude of valuable uses. I believe that it has powerful blood cleansing properties and is valuable for circulatory disorders and conditions resulting in too much acidity.

Lemon has the remarkable ability in aiding the body to eliminate excess crystals and uric acid that if left untreated, could lead to pain and inflammation of the joints, rheumatoid arthritis, muscle damage, and stone-forming material in the kidneys. It has the ability to dissolve kidney stones and is frequently selected by cats for this purpose, a condition that is so common in many cats.

Salvatore writes in his book *'The Complete Guide to Aromatherapy'* 'it improves the functioning of the digestive system, counteracts acidity in the body and makes the stomach more alkaline'.[10]

Lemon clears the mind aiding concentration. In a Japanese study it was found to reduce typing errors by 54% when vapourised into the air.[26] It therefore may be of use for animal training.

Lemons are renowned for their antibacterial properties and their ability to stimulate the production of white blood cells, thus supporting the immune system. This makes lemon essential oil a very useful remedy for related coughs and winter chills. Dr Valnet writes: 'A low dilution of 0.2% lemon essential oil will kill the Diphtheria bacilli in 20 minutes.'[8] Lemon oil is also haemostatic (stops bleeding).

Caution: Do not use undiluted. Photo-reactive.

APPLICATION AND DILUTIONS. Refer to section on administering the oils

Condition	Topical	Oral	Inhalation	Water Bucket
Uplifting **Kidney stones** **Uric / lactic acid** **Immuno-stimulant** **hormone regulator** **Cleansing**		Add 5-7 drops to 5ml base oil	Diluted or undiluted.	Add 3-6 drops to water bowl / bucket

LEMONGRASS
Cymbopogon citratus

Non-toxic, non-irritant
Shelf life: short / moderate

> **Uses**
> Fungal and bacterial infections
> Disorders of the large intestine

Despite its name and its aroma, Lemongrass is not a citrus oil and it is not photo-reactive. It is uplifting and cleansing to the body, mind and spirit and is popular with most mammals.

Lemongrass is a powerful antifungal remedy. Its antiseptic properties help to protect animals from contagious disease.

Lemongrass stimulates the parasympathetic nervous system, aiding digestion and disorders that affect the large intestine (colon). The analgesic action of myrcene, a constituent found in lemongrass, has been confirmed[28].

APPLICATION AND DILUTIONS. Refer to section on administering the oils

Condition	Topical	Oral	Inhalation	Water Bucket
Disorders of the Large intestine		Add 5-7 drops to 5ml base oil	Diluted or undiluted	
Fungal/bacterial infections	Apply undiluted directly on affected area or add to aloe vera gel	as above	as above	

LIME
Citrus aurantifolia

Non-toxic, slight dermal irritant, photo-reactive
Shelf life: short

> **Uses**
> Uplifting
> Fungal and bacterial infections
> Cleansing / liver function

Lime can be distilled or cold pressed but it is the cold pressed oil that is used in animal therapy.

Lime is considered to be anticoagulant, antiseptic and possibly antiviral, so together with its photo - reactive properties, it would be an appropriate oil to offer equines with sarcoids and possibly also other animals with tumours.

Lime is an oil that uplifts the body, mind and spirit. Its primary use is for cleansing the blood and supporting liver function, as well as aiding digestion.

Caution: Cold pressed lime oil is highly photo-reactive.

APPLICATION AND DILUTIONS. Refer to section on administering the oils

Condition	Topical	Oral	Inhalation	Water Bucket
Uplifting Cleansing / liver function		Add 5-7 drops to 5ml base oil	Diluted or undiluted	
Fungal/bacterial infections	Apply to affected area in aloe vera gel	as above	as above	

LINDEN BLOSSOM nature identical
Tilia cordata

Non-toxic, non-irritant
Shelf life: long

> **Uses**
> Physical trauma / abuse
> Lifts heavy emotions

The nature of the oil is predominantly masculine. Linden blossom lifts heavy emotions and helps relieve nervous tension. It is invaluable where animals that have suffered physical trauma or where there has been a history of abuse. Along with angelica root, rose, yarrow and arnica, linden blossom would be a much needed oil for those who work with rescue animals. It is not unusual for it to stimulate an emotional physical release; the results can be dramatic.

The linden blossom used in Animal Aromatics is nature identical, it is a golden brown and has a similar consistency to sandalwood. The linden absolute, which is relatively solid and dark brown is not so often selected by animals and does not, in my experience offer such dramatic results, even though it is of natural rather than synthetic origin.

APPLICATION AND DILUTIONS. Refer to section on administering the oils

Condition	Topical	Oral	Inhalation	Water Bucket
Lifts heavy emotions **Nervous tension** **Physical abuse**		Add 5-10 drops to 5ml base oil	Diluted or undiluted.	A couple of drops

MARJORAM, SWEET
Origanum majorana

Non-toxic, non-irritant
Shelf life: moderate

> **Uses**
> Comforting / grief
> Muscle rubs / warming / Antispasmodic
> Hormones (male) / aggression / excessive mounting

Sweet marjoram is suited to conditions associated with grief and loneliness offering comfort and easing anxiety.

It has strong antispasmodic properties and is renowned for warming and easing stiff joints, tense muscles and hard sinews. Sweet marjoram can also be beneficial for disorders of the digestive tract, such as colic and diarrhoea and it can affect the male hormonal system by balancing excessive sexual desire.

Sweet marjoram should not to be confused with Spanish marjoram, *Thymus mastichina*, which has a high 1,8-cineole content and is used for respiratory and joint disorders.

APPLICATION AND DILUTIONS. Refer to section on administering the oils

Condition	Topical	Oral	Inhalation	Water Bucket
Grief **Aggression** **Excessive sexual excitability**		Add 5-7 drops to 5ml base oil	Diluted or undiluted	
Muscle rubs / warming/ anti-spasmodic	Add 15-20 drops to 150ml watery aloe vera gel	as above	as above	

MUGWORT, GREAT
Artemisia arborescens

Non-toxic, non-irritant
Shelf life: moderate / long

> **Uses**
> Skin allergies
> Lung (respiratory): allergies
> Skin: thrush
> Laminitis

Great mugwort is characterised by its greenish-blue colour and should not be confused with mugwort *(Artemisia herba alba)*, a clear liquid essential oil that is considered toxic amongst aromatherapists due to its high ketone content. Ketones are also present in great mugwort but to a much lesser extent.

Allergies and laminitis

Constituents found in great mugwort make it a powerful antihistaminic, and as such invaluable in the treatment of allergy-related disorders, especially those of the skin, respiratory system and laminitis. In cases where the condition is less severe, the animal will often select German chamomile, which like great mugwort, contains sesquiterpenes.

Thrush

The use of great mugwort on equine thrush can be effective and more compatible with some horses than the commonly used tea tree oil. The tea tree oil is however more readily available. Manuka is another good choice.

APPLICATION AND DILUTIONS. Refer to section on administering the oils

Condition	Topical	Oral	Inhalation	Water Bucket
Thrush: equine	Apply a few drops to the affected area 2 x daily then daily or as needed		Diluted or undiluted	
Skin: allergy	Add 5-10 drops to 150ml gel, Apply to the affected area 1-2 x daily or as needed		as above	
Lung: allergy	Dilute as for oral. Dab onto nostrils	Dilute 3-5 drops in 5ml of base oil	as above	
Laminitis		as above	as above	

NUTMEG
Myristica fragrans

Non-toxic, slight dermal irritant
Shelf life: long

Uses
Scattered energy
Unpredictable
Digestion / diarrhoea
Blood stimulant

Scattered energy / unpredictable
Nutmeg is usually selected by animals with scattered energy, or those that are unpredictable, sometimes being calm and then without reason over-excitable or out of control. If nutmeg is selected, also offer vetiver, as these two oils very often seem to be selected by the animal as a pair.

Nutmeg is considered to be euphoric and vetiver, which is extracted from the roots, helps the animal to become more grounded and focused. Together they seem to have a balancing effect.

Even though nutmeg is considered non-toxic in small amounts, in large doses it can be hallucinogenic. This is believed to be largely due to the myristicin and elemicin found in nutmeg, which metabolise into hallucinogenic substances. Research showed mind-altering effects similar to those obtained by drinking alcohol[29].

Digestion / diarrhoea
Nutmeg is known for its properties in stimulating the blood, the digestive system and for alleviating diarrhoea. Scientists investigated the effect of eugenol, a constituent found in nutmeg oil, for the treatment of diarrhoea and found that it lowered intestinal fluid accumulation and showed anti-inflammatory activity[30].

APPLICATION AND DILUTIONS. Refer to section on administering the oils

Condition	Topical	Oral	Inhalation	Water Bucket
Scattered energy Unpredictable	Add 5-10 drops to 5ml of fixed oil. Apply to paws, poll / forehead or nostrils	Add 5-10 drops in 5ml of fixed oil	Diluted or undiluted	
Digestion		Add 3-4 drops in 5ml of base oil, or gel. Shake well	as above	

ORANGE BLOSSOM / NEROLI

Citrus aurantium ssp. *aurantium*

Non-toxic, non-dermal irritant
Shelf life: moderate / long

Uses

Sadness manifesting in the heart
Separation
Emotional exhaustion / depression
Deep emotional pain
Digestive disorders of an emotional origin

Neroli was the name given to orange blossom after an Italian princess, Anna Maria of Nerola, who wore it as a perfume. It is extracted from the flowers of the bitter orange tree; the white blossoms with their thick fleshy petals are hand picked and then distilled.

Look for a sweet aroma with a bitter undertone of orange scented flowers. Some suppliers succumb to the temptation of adulterating neroli with orange essential oil, which is an inexpensive oil, thus gaining considerable profit while providing an inferior oil. True neroli made from the orange blossoms commands a high price that is comparable to other precious oils, such as rose otto and jasmine.

Sadness taken to the heart / separation

Neroli has a powerful psychological effect, offering a feeling of emotional harmony. It is predominantly used where there is sadness due to the loss or separation of a companion, either human or animal, or in cases of too-early separation from the mother. Such experiences lie dormant in the memory and can very often be the root cause of an illness later on in life. Animals will also almost always select neroli when they have lost the will to recover, or even to live.

I have noticed that when animals select neroli, their breathing initially changes on inhalation to a shallow but fast breath. Neroli may also cause the animal to whimper - perhaps releasing a memory deep within the heart.

The Doctrine of Signatures would regard oranges as resembling the sun. As with most citrus species, bitter orange trees demand a high light intensity for their growth. Thus one could say that neroli is akin to 'distilled sunlight in a bottle'

Digestive disorders of an emotional origin

The antispasmodic action of neroli calms the digestive system, making it useful for anxiety related disorders such as stress-related diarrhoea and colic. Neroli is also used to heal small broken blood vessels below the surface of the skin, and to promote cell growth.

APPLICATION AND DILUTIONS. Refer to section on administering the oils

Condition	Topical	Oral	Inhalation	Water Bucket
Separation / loss Sadness **Digestive problems of an emotional origin**	Dab on to poll / forehead / chest, paws or stroke with neroli water on the hands, gently over the body	Add 2-3 drops to 5ml of water or a fixed oil	Diluted or undiluted.	Add 3-5 drops to a bucket or bowl of water

PEPPERMINT
Mentha x piperita

Non-toxic, slight dermal irritant
Shelf life: moderate / long

Uses
Inflammation to tendons & muscles
Aches and sprains
Nerve damage
Circulation stimulant
Respiratory tract disorders
Digestive disorders
Lethargy / boredom / lack of concentration
Lack of confidence
Burns / overheating

Peppermint oil is frequently selected by horses. Most people believe that this interest is due to the association that it has with mint-flavoured sweets. However, I am inclined to think that it is the peppermint essential oil found in the confectionery that the horse is attracted to, not the sweets. This may be demonstrated by offering a mint in one hand and the oil in the other and observing which the horse chooses. In my experience it has always been the peppermint essential oil. I also know of a horse that loved the smell of peppermint sweets, but once in his mouth he quickly spat them out, while he eagerly licked the peppermint oil.

Peppermint is also popular with cats, it supports digestive function and is generally stimulating to both mental activity and bodily function. A few drops may be added to powdered clay for fleas. Numerous successful research projects have been carried out on peppermint oil, mainly focused on its analgesic properties and its effect on IBS (irritable bowel syndrome).[31] As a result, drugs such as Mintec have been formulated, based on the constituents found in peppermint oil.

Inflammation to tendons and muscles / aches and sprains
Peppermint has valuable anti-inflammatory properties when applied to sprains and similar conditions associated with tendon and muscle damage. Its anti-inflammatory properties are used where there is heat but where the skin is not broken; broken inflamed skin tissue would need an azulene-based oil such as yarrow. Peppermint offers both hot and cold sensations. The warmth of the oil causes the muscles to relax and the cold controls the blood flow to the area, thus having an anti-inflammatory effect. The principles of hot and cold are used in many commercial pain-killing medications.

Circulation / nerve stimulant
Peppermint is indicated where the circulation has been impaired and it is especially useful for horses on box rest or for animals with restricted movement (juniper or celery seed may also be needed for fluid retention and arthritic conditions). Peppermint is a powerful stimulant to the central nervous system, making it one of the most useful remedies for nerve damage. It is also used for lack of concentration and boredom. Research on the topical efficacy of peppermint oil (10% peppermint oil in ethanol) has shown it to be successful in the treatment of tension headaches[32].

Respiratory tract
Many horses have much demand put on their lungs so it is not surprising that peppermint is

one of the most sought after oils by the equine. It offers valuable antibacterial properties while also having the ability to stimulate the functioning and cleansing of the respiratory tract.

Digestion Black's Veterinary Dictionary states 'Peppermint water is added to digestive mixtures to prevent colic and flatulence [20]'. Peppermint is renowned for its therapeutic effect on the small and large intestines, due to its antispasmodic, anti-inflammatory and stimulating properties. Its effect in alleviating the symptoms of colic have been outstanding.

Itchy Skin

Peppermint does the job when it comes to itchy skin. Not only does it help numb the nerve receptors, alleviating the itch but it cools the skin dispersing the heat. Apply it in a gel, if an antihistemic is needed, also offer German chamomile.

Burns

Peppermint in my experience is by far the most effective oil for burns. It appears to take the pain and heat out of the burn almost instantly, and results in remarkably rapid healing.

APPLICATION AND DILUTIONS. Refer to section on administering the oils

Condition	Topical	Oral	Inhalation	Water Bucket
Respiratory tract	Add 10-20 drops to 150ml of a loose gel. Apply to windpipe / neck	Add 5-10 drops to 5ml fixed oil. A 50% dilution may be needed	Diluted or undiluted	Add 5-10 drops to a bowl or bucket of water
Aches and sprains anti-inflammatory Circulation stimulant Nerve damage	Add 20-40 drops to 150ml of gel. Other oils may also be needed. Apply 1-2 x daily or as needed	as above	as above	as above
Boredom Lethargy Lack of concentration	Apply a dab diluted to poll / forehead or paws	as above	as above	as above
Digestive problems		as above	as above	as above
Burns Over heating	Apply undiluted to burn. Add 10-20 drops to 150ml aloe gel, apply to heated areas			
Fleas Toothpaste	Add a few drops to powdered green clay for fleas. It can also be used for brushing dogs teeth			

PINK LOTUS, ABSOLUTE
Nelumbo nucifera

Non-toxic, non-irritant
Shelf life: long

> **Uses**
> Calming
> Balancing

This beautiful flower blooms on the waters' surface at dawn when innocence fills the air. The pink lotus flower is sacred in India and the Far East where it symbolises spirituality, fertility and love. It is from the petals that the fragrance is extracted.

Behavioural problems: calming and focusing
As it slowly opens its petals the pink lotus flower emits a fragrance that balances the chakras, giving a sense of patience and calmness for the new day. With its roots anchored in the water, it suggests that its signature is to attach the spirit to earth and focus it.

Pink lotus is probably, together with rose otto, one of the most popular oils with all animals, especially cats. It is often selected when the behavioural problem doesn't really fit into any one particular category.

The kidneys
As the pink lotus lives in water it would suggest that the oil may support the kidneys which are related to fear.

APPLICATION AND DILUTIONS. Refer to section on administering the oils

Condition	Topical	Oral	Inhalation	Water Bucket
Calming / focusing		Add 5-7 drops to 5ml base oil	Diluted or undiluted.	

ROSE
Rosa damascena

Non-toxic:, non-irritant
Shelf life: long

> **Uses**
> Past abuse / trauma / unwanted memories
> Issues an animal may have inherited
> Anger / resentment - associated with the liver
> Emotional wounds / rejection
> Nurturing
> Hormone balancing (female)
> Birthing

Therapeutic associations with the rose stretch back into the past, crossing religious, cultural and geographical boundaries. The rose is thought to be one of the most evolved of all plant species, its oil containing two to three times more constituents than most other plant oils. There are approximately 250 species of rose, and over 10,000 different hybrid varieties. However, only three species are commonly used in aromatherapy: *Rosa gallica* (French), *Rosa centifolia* (Cabbage), and *Rosa damascena* (Damask).

The Bulgarian Damask rose is considered to be the finest quality and is also known as the Holy Rose, shown around the Virgin Mary when she appeared to St Bernadette at Lourdes. The White rose, *R. damascena* var. *alba* is also Bulgarian. Rose otto is a clear volatile oil that is extracted by steam distillation. Thirty flower-heads are required to yield one drop of otto, which is reflected in its cost; an inexpensive rose otto must be doubted because it is not possible to produce it cheaply. Rose otto congeals at $15°C$, but the warmth from hands on the bottle or putting it against the body will soon bring it back into liquid form. Rose absolute produces a thickish orange liquid that is extracted by solvent extraction, giving it a higher yield and therefore a much lower price than the otto.

Make sure that both rose otto and rose absolute are offered to the animal. Rose otto is considered the purer in quality and is selected much more frequently than the absolute. However, the components are different and so both have individual properties to offer. In general I have found that younger animals and those that need a gentle release, respond more often to the rose absolute.

Past abuse / trauma / unwanted memories / issues an animal may have inherited
Rose otto is the most frequently selected of all the remedies by all species, but is not often needed for long periods of time, usually a matter of days, or even just a sniff to aid the release of a trauma. In many respects rose is a difficult oil to use; possibly because it appears to aid in the release of trauma within the memory.

Rose otto is also selected where there are feelings of anger and resentment which originate in the heart, but are manifested in the liver. The rose will help to dissipate the anger and reunite the animal with peace and love.

Rose evokes feelings of warmth and comfort, soothing emotions such as anger and resentment. Gabriel Mojay writes in his book Healing the Spirit ' rose brings warmth to a soul grown cold through abuse or hurt, rose oil can touch the deepest despair, restoring the trust that makes it possible to love again'.[33]

As animals cannot verbalise their trauma or resentment, they very often respond incredibly well to essential oils for their release, especially rose otto. Essential oils appear to be a silent language where communication is through messages contained within their molecules. As with people, not all animals want to face their past, especially all in one go. So you may need to take extra time with rose working gently and slowly with your animal. If your animal chooses to lick it off your hand that is fine too, either in its diluted or undiluted state.

It is important to watch the animal very carefully when offering rose oil, the slightest flare of a nostril or an unusual stillness could be a positive sign, which may be all that is required. If it is felt that rose should be needed but you are unsure if you are getting a response to indicate it is wanted, leave several drops in a bucket of water in the stable over night, with fresh water also available. The next morning you will most likely find that some will have been drunk. This way the remedy can then be selected in the animals own time, with its fragrance in its aura, offering a gentle release. If you are working with a dog then put a few drops of rose oil in a bowl of water and gently stroke its body with the rose water on your hands. This method can be applied to all species that are able to be touched. When working with rose oil, also offer yarrow as it helps aid protection/support and emotional release.

Balancing female cycles

Rose otto is used more frequently than the absolute for balancing hormones. It will help to bring animals into season and halt prolonged seasons, while also calming mares that are overly marish. The effects of this oil can be seen remarkably quickly for such conditions. A few sniffs of rose otto has also been seen to normalise many weeks of swollen nipples in a young dog within a couple of days. If an animal seems irritable in or around the time she comes into season, also try offering vanilla. You may also want to try offering clary sage, *Salvia sclarea* and geranium, *Pelargonium graveolens*.

Birthing

Most newborns and mothers are keen to inhale the aroma of rose at the time of birth. For the mother it will help regulate and balance the body and the newborn benefits from clearing any trauma from the birth, including issues that they may have brought with them into the world.

APPLICATION AND DILUTIONS Rose. Refer to section on administering the oils

Condition	Topical	Oral	Inhalation	Water Bucket
Female: Balancing cycles	Use undiluted or diluted. Dab onto paws, chest, poll / forehead or stroke hands with rose on gently over the body	Add 2-3 drops of otto or 4-5 drops of absolute to 5ml of water	Diluted or undiluted	Add 1-2 drops in a bowl or 3-5 drops in a bucket of water
Past abuse / trauma Unwanted memories Issues an animal may have been born with	as above		as above	as above
Birthing			as above	Add 5-10 drops in a bowl and apply to tears and affected areas

ROSEMARY
Rosmarinus officinalis

Non-toxic, generally non-irritant
Shelf life: moderate

Uses
Circulation stimulant / muscular stiffness
Coat conditioner / general tonic
Respiratory disorders
Aids concentration use for apathy
Supports confidence / self worth
Mental stimulant

Rosemary is not frequently selected by animals but it may be useful for certain conditions.

Circulation stimulant / muscles
Rosemary is an invigorating circulatory stimulant and a cleanser of the blood. It will act as a general tonic and invigorate bodily functions, making it useful for muscle rubs during travel, before and after endurance work and during box rest. Its warming qualities can also be used as a comforting muscle rub for ageing animals.

Coat conditioner / respiratory
Rosemary will help give shine to a dull coat, and helps to open clogged pores. It is used for coughs where the conditions are cold and damp and has also been used to treat chronic respiratory problems.

Concentration / confidence / self worth
Rosemary inspires feelings of confidence, it is suited to the individual that lacks self worth from experiencing emotional coldness. Its stimulating properties on the mind make it a useful remedy for apathy and mental fatigue. The Romans used to wear rosemary round their heads to aid the memory when they were studying. It may therefore aid in the training of animals.

APPLICATION AND DILUTIONS. Refer to section on administering the oils

Condition	Topical	Oral	Inhalation	Water Bucket
Coat conditioner	Add 10-15 drops to 100ml shampoo base	Add 5-10 drops to 5ml of base oil	Diluted or undiluted	
Lungs	Add 10-20 drops to 200ml of watery gel. Apply to the windpipe or chest	As for above	as above	Add 5-10 drops in a bowl or bucket of water
Stimulant and general tonic	Add 10-20drops to 150ml of watery gel. Apply where needed	As for above	as above	As for above
Supports concentration	Dab undiluted or diluted onto poll / forehead	As for above	as above	

SANDALWOOD
Santalum album

Non-toxic, non dermal-irritant
Shelf life: long

Uses
Upper respiratory infection
Dry flaky skin
Conjunctivitis
Urinary
Ear infections
Obsessive worry / fear
Soothing / comforting / calming

The bulk of sandalwood oil comes from India. It is distilled from the heartwood or roots of trees that are over 30 years old. Sandalwood dates back through time; its uses are amongst the longest recorded, over a period of four thousand years. Several species of sandalwood are available such as *Santalum rubrum,* which grows in Australia and the Pacific Islands. However, none appear to have the equal medicinal value for the mind, as *Santalum album*.

Sandalwood is a popular oil with many animals, especially rabbits. It is a heavy essential oil and does not mix well in water.

Upper respiratory infection
Sandalwood has a pronounced action on the mucus membranes. It has been seen to kill strains of *Staphylococci* and *Streptococci* bacteria[25], and is useful in treating various upper respiratory infections.

Dry flaky skin
The skin and the lungs are both organs of respiration and it is frequently found that the oils used for these two organs overlap. Sandalwood works well for many skin disorders, especially skin that is dry and flaky.

Conjunctivitis / urinary and ear infections
Sandalwood is in all respects a very gentle oil. Its low volatility means that in dilution it does not sting if applied near the eyes and it appears to be effective in combating infections to the eyes. It is an invaluable treatment for conjunctivitis.

In Chinese medicine, the kidneys and bladder govern the ears - the areas where sandalwood has an affinity. I compare sandalwood not to a broad spectrum antibiotic but to one that has specific use in combating infection to the kidneys, bladder, ears and eyes. Sandalwood is selected frequently by animals with ear and urinary tract problems. It plays a powerful role in helping the body fight infection and is invaluable for such treatment. For these conditions the animal usually chooses to take it either orally or by inhalation. In the case of kidney/bladder problems, it can also be applied under the belly inbetween the back legs, where the skin is exposed.

Soothing, comforting and calming
Sandalwood works on the behavioural response in a very similar way to that of frankincense. In some cultures it is still used to anoint the dead and to carry the soul into the next life. Sandalwood comforts the body, mind and spirit while easing fears. It is also indicated for obsessive worry.

APPLICATION AND DILUTIONS Sandalwood Refer to section on administering the oils

Condition	Topical	Oral	Inhalation	Water Bucket
Upper respiratory infection		Add 10-20 drops to 5ml base oil	Diluted or undiluted	
Skin: Dry flaky	Add 10-20 drops to 150ml gel or shampoo base	as above	as above	
Behavioural: Soothing Comforting Calming	Apply diluted or undiluted to poll / forehead, chest or paws	as above	as above	
Kidney / Bladder: Urinary infections	Add 10-20 drops to 5ml of base oil. Apply inbetween back legs where skin is exposed	as above	as above	
Conjunctivitis & Ear infections	Add 3-4 drops to 100ml of warm water. Immerse cotton wool, squeeze out excess water and clean eyes or ears. Apply as needed	as above	as above	

Caution

Normally, essential oils are not applied directly in or around the eye. If eye irritation occurs, the standard industry advice is to rinse with copious amounts of water. In practice, many people find that vegetable oil provides swift relief if applied to the eye with a cotton pad.

SEA BUCKTHORN, CO$_2$ extract
Hippophae rhamnoides

Non-toxic, non dermal irritant
Shelf life: long

Uses
Cancer
Gastric and duodenal ulcers
Liver disease
Skin disorders: palmitoleic acid (a fatty acid) found in sea buckthorn is a component of the skin*
Tissue regeneration
Immune function
UV blocking

Sea buckthorn is popular with all animals. The ancient Greeks fed sea buckthorn to their racehorses to make their coat shine, which gave rise to its Latin name Hippophae, meaning 'horse shine'. Sea buckthorn is mainly produced in China and is CO$_2$ extracted from the berries and the seeds.

Protection against free radicals
The brightly coloured orange/red plant pigment is a visible sign that the fruit is rich in carotenes that protect the plant from free radical damage. Once ingested, carotene offers the same protection to mammals - another indication of our relationship with plants.

Protection against infectious diseases / cell renewal / healthy skin and coat
Beta carotene is converted into vitamin A by the body. Excessive amounts of vitamin A can be toxic but beta carotene will only manufacture the amounts needed. Vitamin A plays an important role in protection against infectious diseases, helping to maintain mucus membranes which form the first line of defence against bacteria, viruses and other irritants. It is necessary for cell renewal, a healthy skin and coat and also supports the functioning of millions of light sensitive structures in the eyes. The berries offer a rich source of flavonoids (antioxidants, antviral, anti-inflammatory).

UV damage and skin cancer
Recent research has shown that recommended amounts of beta carotenes may shield the skin from sun damage.[34] Additionally, carotenoids, have been shown to help protect against certain types of skin cancer.[35]

High in vitamin C
Sea buckthorn berries are second only to rosehips in the amount of vitamin C they contain. They are also rich in other vitamins including B1, B2, K and P and have a remarkably high content of essential fatty acids (EFAs).

Oxidation / free radicals
Free radicals cause damage to cells through a process known as oxidation. Over time this damage can lead to wear and tear and the ageing of cells, in some cases this can lead to cancer and heart problems. Antioxidents counteract the effects of free-radicals.

APPLICATION AND DILUTIONS Sea buckthorn Refer to section on administering the oils

Condition	Topical	Oral	Inhalation	Water Bucket
Cancer **Ulcers** **Liver disorders** **Skin disorders**		Undiluted or diluted at 50%		
Tissue regeneration **Immune function** **UV blocking**	Apply undiluted or in 50% aloe gel	as above		

SEAWEED ABSOLUTE
Fucus vesiculosus

Non-toxic, non-irritant
Shelf life: long

Uses
Run down / loss of condition
Ageing and young animals
Immune stimulant / tumours / cancer
Toxic conditions / vaccine reactions
Impaired movement
Degenerative disorders
Wounds and abscesses - especially cats
Colic / liver dysfunction
Thyroid conditions
Nerve dysfunction
Laminitis

Seaweed is divided into four groups according to its colour: green, brown, red and blue-green.

The name kelp usually refers to the brown variety found in salt water and *Fucus vesiculosus* is commonly known as 'bladder wrack' on account of its bulbous bladder shape with urethra like tubes extending from it. Using the principles of the Doctrine of Signatures, it could then possibly be helpful with bladder disorders. The seaweed used in animal aromatics is a very concentrated viscous dark green extract that is obtained by solvent extraction from the bladder wrack species. The explanation for its powerful effect on animal disease is outlined below.

Kelp plants absorb vitamins and minerals from the sea while their fronds take in energy from sunlight. Using the process of photosynthesis, kelp provides abundant minerals, nutrients and trace elements; ten to twenty times the amount found in land-plants.

The concentrated liquid seaweed extract provides a potent remedy as it is absorbed readily into the blood stream via the buccal and sublingual membranes in the mouth, whereas dried seaweed preparations need to first enter the gut where enzymes begin to break it down, lessening its potency. Seaweed is an excellent remedy for run-down and ageing animals and offers an abundance of nutrients that older animals may find difficult to absorb from food.

Seaweed would be highly recommended in the tack room or the home as its use is so versatile. It is selected by many species for a vast variety of problems and has been invaluable in cases of colic, laminitis, toxic conditions and when movement has been impaired. It is the number one remedy for treating wounds on cats together with green clay.

Seaweed is made up of the following:
Calcium: For bones, teeth and the immune system.
Iron: For anaemia. Helps the body absorb and utilise vitamins.
Iodine: For its antiseptic properties, cuts and bruises and hypothyroid disorders. It also helps to neutralise radioactive materials.
Sulphur: Purifies the blood. Combats skin and hair disorders. Antibacterial and anti-fungal.
Silica: For hooves, bones and coat. It is present in almost every tissue and is essential for cell

growth. It is especially concentrated in hair, nails and connective tissue such as the skin and has an important roll in the synthesis of bone cartilage and collagen.

Magnesium: For nerve and muscle function. It is responsible for the production of ATP (Adenosine triphosphate) within the cell. It also helps control calcium in bones and teeth, rather than allowing it to filter into the blood and kidneys.

Phosphorus: For bones and also protects cells, assisting the activity of nutrients, hormones and chemicals.

Potassium: To help regulate body fluids and form electrolytes. Essential in conducting nerve impulses.

Copper: To help to metabolise iron - a deficiency may cause loss of pigmentation.

Zinc: Wounds, skin disorders and hair loss. Immune stimulant. Enhances sense of smell and taste. Supports the nervous system.

Selenium: Supports liver function. Plays a major roll in thyroxine metabolism and reproductive health.

Kelp also contains: protein, sodium, amino acids, fibre, carbohydrates, essential fatty acids and vitamins A, B1, B2, B12, folic acid, niacin, C, D, E and K, beta carotene and also trace amounts of arsenic. At a time before World War II arsenic was used in trace amounts in veterinary practice to expel worms in the horse.

Animals grazed on land fertilised with kelp have benefited from healthier skin, hooves and coat, and in cattle an increased milk production.

Immune stimulant / detoxifying

Seaweed is a powerful immune stimulant and is indicated where the immune system has been weakened. Kelp extracts have been seen to fight against certain cancers[36] and associated infections.

Researchers have shown seaweed to be important in the fight against cancer because of its anti-tumour activity[36]. This may be one explanation for the low rates of cancers in Japan. People living on Oki Island, where there is an abundance of seaweed in the diet, have the longest life expectancy in Japan.

Alginic acid found in kelp has been shown to give protection against radiation burns. Dr. Tanka, a research scientist at McGill University in Canada, showed that alginic acid binds with heavy metals such as cadmium, mercury and lead, forming an insoluble gel-like salt, which is eliminated from the body tissues and prevents their reabsorption into the blood[37]. He also reported that sodium alginate, a polysaccharide (starch) found in brown seaweed such as kelp and kombu, can remove radioactive material from the body. Kelp appears to have the natural ability to counteract chronic poisons and may therefore be useful where there has been long-term medication or adverse reactions to vaccines. Green clay and seaweed make a powerful poultice with incredible drawing properties.

Seaweed is also beneficial to the glands and is indicated for disorders such as Cushing's disease, caused by a benign tumour on the pituitary gland, resulting in an over-production of corticosteroid hormones and secondary laminitis.

Impaired movement / laminitis / degenerative disorders
The sea has continuous activity and seaweed is indicated for disorders that involve lack of movement such as laminitis, arthritis and navicular, even colic. Seaweed maintains the elasticity of the blood vessel walls while drawing poisons out of the cells, improving osmotic exchanges and elimination of wastes. The selenium found in kelp also helps to support the liver and the blood.

Wounds and abscesses
Seaweed is excellent for the treatment of wounds as it contains iodine, sulphur and zinc which all play an important role in the healing process. It helps to draw foreign matter from both wounds and abscesses, leaving them clean and disinfected. Together with powdered green clay it is one of the few remedies that can be applied to a cat for such afflictions. The results from treating wounds on cats with seaweed have been very encouraging.

Intestinal problems
Seaweed as an anticoagulant. Its anti-inflammatory and detoxifying properties make it useful in cases of colic, often rapidly alleviating symptoms. *Black's Veterinary Dictionary* states that seaweed 'acts as a digestive tonic by stimulating the muscles of the alimentary canal[20]'.

Contraindication
Ingestion of bladder wrack is normally contraindicated in cases of hyperthyroidism, pregnancy and lactation. However hyperthyroid cats appear to select seaweed extract and often ingest it, perhaps suggesting that if the thyroid is out of balance it will help to correct it. If there are no problems with the thyroid and the animal is forced to ingest it with its food then perhaps it will become problematic.

Oriental medicine
In China seaweed is used to moisten and to cool and soothe inflammations especially in the lungs and throat (coughing) and in conditions of asthma. Seaweed is associated with the Water Element, regulating fluids and supporting the kidneys, while also alleviating liver stagnancy.

Behavioural
Inhaling the sea air clears the mind of confusion installing a sense of peace, while cleansing the body, mind and spirit. The same applies when inhaling seaweed.

APPLICATION AND DILUTIONS Seaweed Refer to section on administering the oils

Condition	Topical	Oral	Inhalation	Water Bucket
Run down **Ageing animals** **Immune disorders** **Toxic conditions** **Liver disorders** **Impaired movement** **Colic**		Add 10-20 drops to 5ml base oil If the animal has a keen interest dilute at 50%	Diluted or undiluted	
Wound healing **Absess** **Puncture wounds**	Apply undiluted to the affected areas. Or add 10-20 drops to 50ml firm aloe vera gel. Apply as needed	as above	as above	

SPEARMINT
Mentha spicata

Non-toxic, non-irritant

Shelf life: moderate

> **Uses**
> Mental stimulant / refreshing
> Chronic obstructive pulmonary disease
> Digestive disorders

Spearmint a member of the peppermint family. It is popular with cats and may be selected in preference to peppermint by young animals and some dogs. In cases of horses with C.O.P.D., spearmint will usually be selected in preference to peppermint.

Spearmint supports digestive function and is generally stimulating to both mental activity and bodily function.

APPLICATION AND DILUTIONS. Refer to section on administering the oils

Condition	Topical	Oral	Inhalation	Water Bucket
Mental stimulant / refreshing **Digestive disorders**		Add 5-15 drops to 5ml base oil or water	Diluted or undiluted	Add 3-6 drops to water bowl / bucket
Respiratory problems	20-30 drops in 150ml watery gel (with other needed oils) applied to the windpipe	as above	as above	as above

SPIKENARD
Nardostachys jatamansi

Non-toxic, non-irritant
Shelf life: long

> **Uses**
> Soothing / calming / comforting

Spikenard, also known as nard, is a member of the valerian family and like valerian, is extracted from the roots. It is an ancient oil that was used by Mary Magdalene to anoint Jesus' feet before the last supper.

It is a great favourite for cats.

Soothing, calming, comforting
Spikenard is often selected by animals that have been through difficult times. The oil seems to penetrate deep into the heart, soothing and comforting the spirit within. Its warmth connects the animal with mother earth, instilling a sense of peace and calm.

Even though its cost is high it is one to have in stock if dealing with troubled animals.

APPLICATION AND DILUTIONS. Refer to section on administering the oils

Condition	Topical	Oral	Inhalation	Water Bucket
Soothing / calming / comforting		Add 5 drops to 5ml base oil	Diluted or undiluted	

TEA TREE
Melaleuca alternifolia

Non-toxic, non-irritant

Shelf life: short

Uses
Viral, fungal and bacterial infections

Wounds / thrush / ringworm

Urinary infections

Insect bites / repellent

Strengthens will power / mind / Confidence

While exploring Australia in the 1770s, Captain Cook gathered the leaves of the Ti-tree to make tea, which is now referred to as tea tree. The infusion seemed to offer his crew good health and resistance to disease. Whether he chose these leaves at random or had some Aboriginal guidance is unclear, but it is known that the Aboriginals have used tea tree for thousands of years, aware of its valuable antiseptic, antibiotic, fungicidal and anti-viral properties.

Tea tree, like eucalyptus is not a popular oil with animals in the Western hemisphere, yet unfortunately, it is found in many commercial animal products. Rarely are these oils selected, however, from time to time these oils are selected and in such cases produce effective results. Perhaps it is more suited to the animals, such as the koala bear that originate from where the plant grows.

There are many species of *Melaleuca* growing in Australia, but the tea tree comes from the trees growing in the river deltas of New South Wales, where it is difficult and dangerous to access. Poisonous spiders and snakes live amongst trees that grow in dark humid low-lying swamps, an ideal environment for viruses and fungi to thrive. Tea tree is yet another example of Mother Nature planting her antidote as the oil will effectively counteract the poisons from these spiders and snakes and also combat viral and fungal afflictions.

Tea tree is a registered medicine in Australia and as such is frequently tested for quality. If cineole reaches levels of over 15% then it is said that the oil becomes caustic to skin. The ideal level is 5% or lower and terpinen 4-ol, an active healing ingredient, must have levels of above 30% for therapeutic use. This is required by the Australian standard for tea tree[39].

Viral / antifungal / antibacterial / wounds
The medicinal uses of tea tree are well documented. In one report it was demonstrated that the bacterial count on unwashed hands was 3000 per 50 cm. After washing in distilled water it dropped to around 2000 per 50 cm then when washed in tea tree the count was less than 3 per 50 cm. Tea tree has also been tested in solution of 4 parts oil to 1000 parts water against virulent organisms such as *Staphylococcus aureus* and *Candida albicans*. The results at 7, 21 and 35 days showed that no growth was detected for any of the organisms. The Medical Journal Australia, of March, 1930 wrote: 'Dirty wounds, such as the result of street accidents, may be washed or syringed out with a 10% tea tree watery lotion, the solvent properties will loosen and bring

away the dirt which is usually ground in and the tissues will remain fresh and retain their natural colour. Dressings dipped in a 2.5% solution may then be applied, changed every 24 hours and healing will readily take place[39].'

Research has also shown tea tree to be an antiseptic bactericide thirteen times stronger than carbolic acid and that in the presence of pus and blood it increased its antiseptic ability by 10-12%[39]. The British Medical Journal stated that tea tree oil is 'a powerful disinfectant, non-poisonous and non-irritating, that has been used successfully in a very wide range of septic conditions[39].'

Ringworm
Ringworm is a fungal infection of the skin, caused by species of *Trichophyton and Microsporum* against which undiluted tea tree is effective, especially when blended with undiluted lavender (larger areas would need these oils to be applied in a gel).

Thrush
Thrush is an infection that affects mainly horses in the frog of the foot. The horn decomposes and forms a black substance that has a characteristic unpleasant odour. The foot must be thoroughly cleaned with water and a stiff brush, then tea tree oil applied.

Urinary infections
Tea tree has a natural antibiotic effect in treating acute urinary infections, as well as helping to stimulate the immune system.

Caution: There have been various reports of strong adverse reactions to tea tree oil, causing temporary paralysis in dogs and cats[40] and severe inflammation with the topical application of the oil to horses' legs. In these cases the quality of the oil must be considered as well as the animals' response to the oil - was the oil offered to the animal before it was applied?

Note: If an animal does not respond to tea tree, try manuka, *Leptospermum scoparium*, which is an excellent alternative. It is sometimes referred to as New Zealand tea tree oil because many of its uses overlap, however it is not a member of the tea tree genus.

APPLICATION AND DILUTIONS Tea tree Refer to section on administering the oils

Condition	Topical	Oral	Inhalation	Water Bucket
Wounds **Thrush** **Ringworm** **Fungal, viral &** **bacterial infections** **Insect bites**	Apply undiluted. For larger areas add 20-30 drops to 50ml firm aloe vera gel	Add 5 drops to 5ml fixed oil	Diluted or undiluted	
Urinary infections		as above	as above	Add 5 drops to a bowl or bucket of water
Immune stimulant		as above	as above	as above

THYME
Thymus vulgaris

Linalol chemotype
Non-toxic, non-irritant
Shelf-life: moderate

Thymus vulgaris

Thymol, Carvacrol chemotypes
Slightly toxic, dermal irritant
Shelf-life: moderate

> ### Uses
> Encourages braveness
> Bacterial infections
> Respiratory infections
> Airborne bacteria
> Worms

There are over 300 different species of thyme. Spanish thyme *(Thymus zygis)* has a high thymol content (50-75%) and is inexpensive, but the most commonly used chemotypes are thymol and carvacrol, extracted from *Thymus vulgaris*. These pungent oils grow at low altitudes close to the Mediterranean Sea. This renders them generally more potent and aggressive than the linalol chemotype which is sweet and herbaceous and found at higher altitudes, giving it a greater alcohol content with less phenolic compounds.

The linalol chemotype is therefore suited to young and sensitive skins and is more of an immunostimulant than an antibacterial. The geraniol chemotype is less frequently used but is indicated for fungal infections.

Avoid selecting thymes by denomination of 'red' or 'white' as these terms mean little in the essential oil industry and can lead to confusion.

Encourages braveness
The Greek word thymon means 'courage'. Roman soldiers would bathe in thyme before entering battle and those departing on crusades would have thyme woven into their scarves. Just a few sniffs of thyme may encourage braveness in an animal.

Bacterial infections
The essential oil of *Thymus zygis* is a stronger antiseptic than hydrogen peroxide or potassium permanganate and has been proven to have a stimulating effect on white corpuscles, boosting the immune system and helping to combat infection.

Thymus vulgaris (carvacrol chemotype) is also used in cases of severe infection. Its undiluted use on infected wounds, together with yarrow is highly recommended. Skin conditions caused by the *Dermatophilus* bacterium, such as mud-fever, also respond well to thyme carvacrol chemotype.

Dr. Valnet, a pioneer of medical aromatherapy has done much to inspire research on the efficacy of essential oils. During the second world war, when supplies of penicillin became unavailable, he used thyme on an amputee to treat gangrene; he found that its effectiveness was comparable to that of the penicillin and that the condition cleared with no further infection or complications[8].

Respiratory infections

Thymus vulgaris (carvacrol and/ or thymol chemotypes) is an excellent broncho-pulmonary and immune stimulant. According to Dr. Valnet 'an aqueous solution of 5% thyme kills typhus bacillus in 2 minutes, colon bacillus in 2-8 minutes, staphylococcus in 4-8 minutes and streptococcus and diphtheric bacillus in 4 minutes'[8].

Airborne bacteria

Thyme is a volatile essential oil that is very effective in killing airborne bacteria. Used in a spray it could help prevent the spread of disease.

Worms

Thyme and garlic have been suggested for the treatment of roundworms, threadworms, hookworms, tapeworms and other intestinal parasites, however, I have had no success for the treatment of worms with essential oils.

APPLICATION AND DILUTIONS. Refer to section on administering the oils

Condition	Topical	Oral	Inhalation	Water Bucket
Wounds / Bacterial infections	Apply to wound undiluted or add 10 drops to gel	Add 5 drops to 5ml base oil	Diluted or undiluted	
Respiratory infections		as above	as above	Add 10 drops to water bucket / bowl
Worms		as above	as above	Add 10 drops to a bucket of water
Courage / Braveness	Add 3-5 drops to 5ml base oil or gel. Dab onto forehead / poll, chest or paws	as above	as above	Add 10 -20 drops to 150ml loose gel, use as a spray. Shake well
Airborne bacteria		as above	as above	

VALERIAN
Valeriana officinalis

Non-toxic, non-irritant
Shelf life: long

> **Uses**
> Relaxing / focusing
> Muscle rub
> Cystitis in cats
> Epilepsy

Valerian is a known sedative, but is not related to valium. Valerian sedates the central nervous system, although it also stimulates digestion and the cardiovascular system. The oil is extracted from the roots, and is very 'grounding'.

Behavioural: relaxing and focusing
Valerian should be offered to animals that are unable to relax or focus; its effects can be immediate. It is a popular oil with all animals especially cats, instilling deep relaxation making it a useful remedy for stress-related cystitis which is common in cats.

You may want to check that your animal is absorbing enough nutrients, especially magnesium, which if lacking can contribute to anxious, nervous or spooky behaviour. If you are in doubt, also offer seaweed and spirulina which are rich in magnesium. Sugars are also a well known cause of excitable, anxious behaviour.

Tense, tight muscles
When added to a gel valerian makes an excellent rub for tense, tight muscles. It is especially effective when used with other oils such as peppermint, wintergreen, marjoram and juniper berry.

Epilepsy
The use of valerian has been suggested for epilepsy.

APPLICATION AND DILUTIONS. Refer to section on administering the oils

Condition	Topical	Oral	Inhalation	Water Bucket
Relaxing / focusing **Cystitis in cats** **Epilepsy**		Add 5 drops to 5ml base oil	Diluted or undiluted	
Muscle rub	Add 10 -15 drops to 150ml watery aloe vera gel			

VANILLA, ABSOLUTE
Vanilla planifolia

Non-toxic, non-irritant
Shelf life: long

> **Uses**
> Comforting
> Irritability / anger
> Nervous tension

Next to saffron and cardamom, vanilla is the world's next most expensive spice. Its fragrance is sweet and warm. The Bourbon vanilla beans generally contain higher amounts of vanillin than the Mexican and Tahiti beans. Vanilla is used both in pharmaceutical products and food flavouring. Its thickish consistency makes it difficult to pour, so a glass rod is often needed.

Vanilla is an incredibly effective oil for irritability especially when relating to female cycles. It is usually taken orally and is popular with many animals, softening anger, instilling relaxation and easing frustration.

Vanilla is thought to induce DNA repair; an example of a naturally occurring chemical that increases the level of DNA repair is vanillin.[41]

APPLICATION AND DILUTIONS. Refer to section on administering the oils

Condition	Topical	Oral	Inhalation	Water Bucket
Comforting Irritability / anger		Add 5-10 drops to 5ml base oil	Diluted or undiluted.	

VETIVER
Vetiveria zizanioides

Non-toxic, non-irritant
Shelf life: long

Uses
Calms / restores
Centres / focus and reconnects
Nurturing / reassuring
Balances sexual excitability
Anaemia
Venous tonic

The vetiver plant is a tall grass, approximately 6ft (2m) high, with a mass of fine spongy roots. It is at home in Southern India, the Himalayan mountains, Sri Lanka and Malaysia, but the finest quality is the bourbon vetiver from the Reunion Islands.

The oil is extracted from the roots of vetiver grass which yields a thickish, dark brown oil that does not pass through the dropper easily, making it difficult to get an exact measurement. In such a case, remove the dropper and pour the oil slowly into the base product.

Unfocussed / ungrounded / over excited / restless
Vetiver offers the reassuring comfort of Mother Earth, bringing a deeper sense of belonging. It sedates yet restores and has a calming, grounding effect, allowing the animal to focus. It is very popular with all animals including cats.

Vetiver very often works in conjunction with nutmeg, especially with horses and if an animal's energy is scattered and unpredictable.

Excessive sexual excitability
Vetiver has an effect on hormonal activity and can help to restore balance in cases of oestrogen and progesterone insufficiency. It also effects the male hormonal system, calming sexual excitability, especially with rigs.

Anaemia / venous tonic
The Doctrine of Signatures would indicate that the roots of a plant are generally associated with nourishment, strength and grounding. This reflects the use of vetiver, which is indicated for anaemia and malabsorption.

Components within vetiver oil have been found to inhibit the binding of vasopressin and therefore to exert a distinct influence on the tone of the blood vessels.

APPLICATION AND DILUTIONS. Refer to section on administering the oils

Condition	Topical	Oral	Inhalation	Water Bucket
Unfocussed Ungrounded Over excited Restless Sexual excitability Anaemia Venous tonic	Use undiluted or diluted. Dab onto nostrils or paws	Add 5-10 drops to 5ml of base oil	Diluted or undiluted.	

VIOLET LEAF, ABSOLUTE
Viola odorata

Oral toxicity unknown, non-dermal irritant
Shelf life: long

Uses
Nervousness
Spooking
New home / yard
Vices: Box walking
Clip-shy
Heart (comforting)

Violet leaf is an absolute made from the leaves of the plant, which produces a rich green liquid with a strong leafy aroma resembling cut cucumbers. The flowers from the plant can also be used to make an absolute, yielding a yellowish green oil, with a sweet floral fragrance, but it offers quite different therapeutic properties.

Some violet leaf oils on the market have been adulterated with spinach, so be sure to purchase it from a trusted supplier. Violet leaf absolute is relatively thick in its consistency and can be quite difficult to dispense through the dropper, especially in cold climates, when you will need to warm the bottle in your hands or against your body to help liquify it. Then remove the dropper and let it drop slowly from the rim of the bottle.

Nervous / new home, yard / insecurity / vices
Violet leaf is a popular remedy with animals, especially dogs and horses that are tense, nervous and spook easily or that have recently moved to a new home or yard. It is also helpful for problems such as box walking and for animals that are clip-shy and those that do not rest easily.

Violet leaf contains salicylic acid, a natural pain-killer, which could possibly also act on the mind, numbing emotional pain. As with all calming essential oils, it will not dull the senses, rather it will help the animal keep in control, maintaining inner strength that would otherwise be depleted or scattered.

Violet leaf can help an animal to be introduced to a new experience. The heart-shaped violet leaves reflect their traditional use, to comfort and strengthen the heart. Its application is normally always oral and some animals will need it undiluted, as in dilution they will never seem to get their required dose, taking 5mls in several licks, only to look for more.

APPLICATION AND DILUTIONS. Refer to section on administering the oils

Condition	Topical	Oral	Inhalation	Water Bucket
Behavioural problems		Add 5-10 drops to 5ml of base. A stronger application is often needed at 50% dilution or undiluted	Diluted or undiluted.	

WINTERGREEN
Gaultheria procumbens

YELLOW BIRCH
Betula alleghaniensis

Oral toxicity, possible skin irritant / inhibits blood clotting

Shelf life: Moderate / long

Uses
Muscular aches / inflammation
Anti-platelet activity
Pain killing / analgesic
Arthritis

There are several types of Birch; yellow birch *Betula alleghaniensis*, Silver birch *Betula pendula* and cherry birch *Betula lenta*, but it is the yellow birch that is used in animal therapy. As with wintergreen, its aroma will be familiar as it is found in many pharmaceutical preparations.

I have written wintergreen and birch together because their properties and effects overlap. They both contain approximately 98% methyl salicylate, which is a derivative of salicylic acid, found in many plants. Medical salicylic compounds are used as analgesics and antipyretics, sold under trade names such as aspirin.

Most aromatherapy publications state that the use of wintergreen and birch should be avoided both internally and externally, as they work in a similar way to aspirin, and also because most of the wintergreen that is available is synthetically produced methyl salicylate. However their use has been invaluable in reducing pain and inflammation.

Muscular aches / inflammation / anti-platelet activity / arthritis / analgesic properties

Both wintergreen and birch have a deep heat, anti-inflammatory and analgesic effect on muscular aches, sprains, tendon injuries and arthritis. They are used in many pharmaceutical preparations and I have found them invaluable for relieving both chronic and acute muscular problems. In general horses seem to select wintergreen more frequently and dogs prefer birch.

Caution: Do not apply wintergreen or birch to open wounds. Both oils thin the blood and are not compatible with anti-coagulant pharmaceutical drugs such as warfarin and aspirin, which can heighten its anticoagulant effect. Methyl salicylate can be absorbed transdermally in sufficient quantities to cause this type of poisoning. If animals are awaiting surgery it will increases the risk of haemorrhage. Salicylates can be dangerous to cats.

APPLICATION AND DILUTIONS. Refer to section on administering the oils

Condition	Topical	Oral	Inhalation	Water Bucket
Muscular strain Pain. Arthritis. Inflammation.	Add 10-15 drops to 150ml gel Apply to affected areas 1-2 x daily or as needed. Its action may be enhanced with oils such as Peppermint, Juniper and yarrow	Add 5 drops to 5ml fixed oil	Diluted or undiluted.	

YARROW
Achillea millefolium

Non-toxic, non-irritant
Shelf life: long

> **Uses**
> Wounds of the body and heart
> Anti-inflammatory -healing to
> Release of trauma from wound
> Repressed anger from a wounded heart
> Over-sensitivity - protector
> (the flowers are grouped together resembling a shield)
> Kidney / Bladder problems

Yarrow can be a confusing oil to purchase, as the Latin name will be the same but the colour and properties can be very different. The amount of chamazulene within yarrow essential oil can vary considerably, ranging from 5.5 - 33%; thus offering a very different oil with very different properties. The 33% oil will be dark blue and rich in chamazulene, while the 5.5% oil will be clear and possibly higher in ketones.

It is the chamazulene that gives yarrow its strong anti-inflammatory, anti-histamine, cell regenerating and analgesic properties. The ketone rich oil, even though it stimulates the formation of tissue and has mucolytic properties, can be potentially neurotoxic. The yarrow described in this book is recognised by its sweet aroma and ink-blue colour, which means it is rich in chamazulene. This chemotype also can have a powerful effect on the emotional / behavioural responses.

Emotional wounds of the heart / wounds of the body / over-sensitivity / emotional release

The psychological use of yarrow complements its ability to treat wounds by helping to release the trauma associated with them. Yarrow is frequently used alongside rose oil to aid the release of past issues. Even though yarrow is a favourite with many animals, it is especially so for horses. This may be due to an inbuilt recognition as yarrow was once used extensively on battlefields to treat the wounds of both man and horse.

The animal selecting yarrow will usually choose to lick it off the hand as well as enjoying inhaling its aroma. Yarrow should be offered when there is emotional or physical sensitivity, as it is a protector to both the body and soul. The flowers from this plant are grouped together and shaped like a shield, signifying their protective use.

Yarrow is in my opinion the most beneficial and effective remedy to apply to a wound. It is an oil to select and offer animals with external inflictions that have damaged or irritated the skin; it is indicated where there is inflammation, heat and where pus is exuding from exposed broken, inflamed tissue. It seems to take the pain and heat out on application - if you cut yourself it is worth trying yarrow and experiencing it for yourself.

The blue colour indicates a cooling effect and yarrow does just that. For conditions where excess heat causes irritation, pain or itchiness such as sweet itch or insect bites, yarrow is a good choice . It is amazing how quickly it takes the itch out of insect bites.

Yarrow is not an oil that is noted for its antibacterial properties, yet when applied to wounds it seems to provide an environment that inhibits the growth of bacteria. Sam Davis who has a section in this book working at a cattery, would easily get an infection at the site of a cat bite if she did not treat it. So she decided to test the yarrow, which she normally dislikes, (except after being bitten when it then becomes appealing). The wound healed with no associated infection! The anti-infectious properties may come from supporting immune responses, rather than acting directly against infective organisms.

On isolated areas such as wounds and insect bites, yarrow is usually more beneficial applied undiluted. When yarrow is dropped onto the affected area you may notice that it completely absorbs into the affliction, while the surrounding area may stain blue. Complete absorption means that more needs to be applied so repeat the process until it stains the area.

Gattefosse noted that essential oils diluted to a degree at which they no longer have any effect on cultures in vitro (a test solution outside the body), still have a clear, rapid and beneficial action in vivo (in the living body).[42] This may account for the effectiveness of yarrow.

Kidneys / bladder

Yarrow is indicated where there is urinary infection which is associated with inflammation and / or emotional trauma. Together with sandalwood, yarrow is the most frequently selected oil for urinary infections.

APPLICATION AND DILUTIONS Yarrow Refer to section on administering the oils

Condition	Topical	Oral	Inhalation	Water Bucket
Wounds: **Pus-filled /** **Inflamed**	Apply several drops undiluted onto the affected area, until the blue stains the wound	Add 5 drops in 5ml of base oil	Diluted or undiluted	
Skin: **Raw / inflamed** **Irritated** **Itchy** **Allergy**	As above or add 10 drops to 50ml aloe vera gel	as above	as above	
Behavioural **Problems**	Dab undiluted or diluted onto nostrils or paws	as above	as above	
Kidney / Bladder	Add 5-7 drops to 10ml base oil, or 50ml aloe gel, apply to belly area in-between back legs where skin is exposed.	as above	as above	
Lungs: Allergies		as above	as above	

YLANG YLANG
Cananga odorata

Non-toxic, possible slight dermal irritant
Shelf life: Moderate / long

> **Uses**
> Offers feelings of self worth / confidence
> Comforting / instills peace
> Balances sexual behaviour (male)
> Aggressive male dominant behaviour
> Epilepsy

The ylang tree is tall, with large, fragrant flowers. The cultivated ylang tree produces a more potent fragrance than the wild variety. Like jasmine, the blossoms need to be harvested and prepared in the early morning hours when their fragrance is at its strongest. There are five different grades of ylang ylang, the most aromatic, preferred by perfumers is ylang ylang extra. The ylang ylang used in animal aromatics is ylang ylang complete which contains a broader range of constituents. Ylang ylang was once known as the poor man's jasmine, however I have found it to be popular with many animals.

Self-worth / confidence / comforting / stable vices / encourages males to cover

Animals that lack confidence, or those that bully others often select ylang ylang. It is also frequently selected by animals that are nervous.

It is thought that ylang ylang contains various constituents, which stimulate the production of endorphins. Its relaxing and hormonal effect can be very effective in encouraging sexual activity, particularly in the male. Animals that are overly aggressive and dominant have also benefited from ylang ylang.

Pathogens

At the beginning of the 20th century two French chemists discovered that ylang ylang was effective against malaria, typhus and infections of the intestinal tract.[10]

Epilepsy

According to Tim Betts of Birmingham University's Neuropsychiatry Clinic, England, ylang ylang oil can be effective for controlling epilepsy, especially when smelled at the onset of a seizure. The majority of patients with epilepsy, given a choice of four or five oils, invariably choose ylang ylang.[43]

APPLICATION AND DILUTIONS. Refer to section on administering the oils

Condition	Topical	Oral	Inhalation	Water Bucket
Behavioural problems	Dab onto paws, poll or forehead	Add 4-7 drops to 5ml of base oil	Diluted or undiluted	
Pthogens		as above	as above	
Epilepsy	Dilute. Dab onto paws, poll or forehead			

first aid

Items for your first aid kit

- Blanket: to use as a stretcher or to cover an animal in shock
- Disposable gloves
- Emergency numbers for veterinary surgeons / note book
- Essential oils and plant extracts (in particular: rose, yarrow, arnica macerated oil, peppermint, carrot seed and aloe vera gel)
- Large bandages, gauze pads, tape, scissors
- Essential oil bottles / jars
- Plastic bag
- Bottled water (for mixing and cleaning)
- Tea towel / cloth
- Thermometer

Basic first aid for conditions that need immediate veterinary attention

Condition	Remedies to offer while waiting for veterinary attention
Colic	Seaweed, peppermint, Roman and German chamomile
Unconscious	Peppermint inhalation
Major bleed - external haemorrhage	Yarrow, rose arnica and carrot seed
Internal haemorrhage	Yarrow and carrot seed
Hyperthermia - heat stroke	Cool towels soaked in peppermint water
Raised temperature / infection: horse	Offer eucalyptus and immune stimulants
Raised temperature / infection: dog	Offer thyme and immune stimulants
Raised temperature / infection: cat	Offer lemon, and immune stimulants
Road traffic accidents	Rose, yarrow, arnica for shock
Poisoning: N.B. cats have a limited ability to metabolise paracetamol, over dose is easy and can be fatal.	Seaweed, charcoal, clay, bread and milk. Do not induce vomiting an hour after poisoning or where corrosive materials have been ingested.
Burns	Peppermint in aloe vera gel, or water applied topically
Electrocution Do not approach the animal until electricity has been turned off	Internal electric burn / radiation - spirulina or seaweed. Arnica, rose and yarrow for shock. Offer internal / external

Check the animal for the following

Condition	Cause	Possible remedies	Cause	Possible remedies
Pale gums	Shock	Arnica, rose, yarrow	Internal bleeding or external bleeding	Carrot seed, yarrow
Blue gums	Lack of oxygen	Make sure airway is clear		
Yellow gums	Possible liver problem	Carrot seed, seaweed		
Dilated pupils	Head injury	Arnica, rose, yarrow, peppermint	Shock Poisoning / drugs	

Caution:
Be careful when offering certain essential oils as they could affect the metabolism of drugs, either exacerbating or reducing their effect. Apply some caution with arnica if medicines other than antibiotics are needed.

An injured animal is unpredictable and may bite, scratch or kick when approached. Use caution and get assistance if necessary. A blanket can be used to cover the head or to restrain a small animal.

Suspected fractures

Keep the animal still and calm
Support and immobilise the fracture.
Offer arnica, rose, yarrow

Serious wounds / injury

Gaping wounds or those over one inch long may need stitching and should be checked by your vet. With horses it is often found that wounds below the knee/hock seem to be more difficult to heal.

Treatment
If blood is spurting out apply a pad of cotton wool or clean cloth and hold or bandage firmly in place. If blood continues to come through the dressing do not remove it but apply another one on top - removing the bandage could disturb newly formed blood clots. Do not bandage too tightly as restricting the circulation for too long can cause further damage to the area. If you are unsure, loosen the bandage but monitor carefully in case bleeding starts again.

Oils to offer
Carrot seed and yarrow - oral / topical / inhalation.

Note: Do not apply essential oils in a base oil to open wounds, as this prevents the wound from drying and attracts dirt.

Problems affecting the nervous system

Oils to offer

Hemp oil	calms the nervous system
Peppermint	stimulates new pathways
St John's wort	virus' effecting nerves / calms
Carrot seed	cell repair

The central nervous system comprises of the brain and the spinal cord. There are many different types of nerve cells, all of which transmit messages to and from the brain. These include the sense of smell, sensations of touch or pain and conscious or unconscious muscular action. Some related disorders include paralysis or loss of sensation to parts of the body, laryngeal hemiplegia (roaring, whistling), wobbler syndrome and stringhalt.

Damaged nerve cells are difficult to repair, instead new neural pathways are formed. These new pathways appear to be encouraged with essential oils such as peppermint. There has been research undertaken recently on the effects of St John's wort on the nervous system, providing very encouraging results. [44]

Internal haemorrhage

It is not always obvious initially that the animal is bleeding internally.

Symptoms could include
Shock
Pale mucus membranes
Difficulty breathing
Vomiting blood
Distension of abdomen
Severe bruising
Blood in the urine or faeces

Oils to offer
Carrot seed and yarrow, orally or by inhalation.

Hyperthermia / heatstroke

Heat exhaustion is commonly seen in short nosed breeds of dog (pug, boxers, bulldogs etc) but can affect any animal.

Symptoms include
Increased body temperature
Excessive panting / salivation
Restlessness / distressed

As the condition deteriorates the animal will become unsteady on its feet and collapse. If it is left untreated it may die.

Treatment
Inform your vet and whilst waiting, wet the animal with cool or tepid peppermint water.

Convulsions / fits

The most common cause of a convulsion is epilepsy or poisoning.

Treatment
Contain the animal in a darkened room
Reduce the amount of noise
Remove objects close to the animal that could hurt them
Stay calm and do not touch the animal
Turn off stimuli such as TV

Oils to offer
Lavender / valerian / ylang ylang / St John's wort macerate, Hemp macerate

The fit may last a few seconds to 5 - 10 minutes or longer. Notify your vet even if the fit has only lasted a short while. Prolonged fitting may need urgent veterinary intervention.

common disorders effecting most species

Many conditions need to have remedies selected and offered that reflect the animals' individual needs. However, where blended formulas are appropriate they will be mentioned in this section. It is important to understand the symptoms and the cause of the problem in order to select the correct oils.

Items for your remedy kit

Glass pots / plastic mixing bottles: 50 - 250 ml
Glass Bottles / 5 ml with droppers - 10 ml with droppers - 50 ml (wide neck for macerates)
Glass stirring rod, plastic spoon
Sticky labels, pen and sellotape to protect written labels against smudging.
Bottle water (for mixing and cleaning)
Essential oils and extracts, macerates, beeswax, Dead Sea mineral mud, clay, spirulina and relevant remedies such as rosehips and devil's claw.

Ringworm

Ringworm is a fungal infection of the skin caused by *Trichophyton* spp. and *Microsporum* spp.

Oils to offer
Lavender and tea tree applied together
Seaweed (the iron in the seaweed is said to be effective against ringworm).

Application
Apply undiluted to the affected area 1-2 x daily or as needed. For larger areas add to aloe vera gel.

Insect bites

Oils to offer
German chamomile, yarrow, lavender, tea tree and peppermint.

German chamomile generally gives the greatest relief. Try it if you get bitten - you will be amazed. It seems to take the pain and itch away almost immediately.

Application
Apply undiluted or in aloe vera gel, as needed. The oils will usually be more effective applied undiluted. Drop the oil onto the bite and allow it to be absorbed. When applying blue oils repeat this until the oil stains the skin. This indicates that the area has taken all that is needed.

Mange

Mange is a caused by Sarcoptic or Demodectic mange mites that live within the skin layers. The condition can cause intense itching and widespread hair loss.

2 drops yarrow
10 drops lavender
6 drops Roman chamomile
1 drop garlic

Add the oils to 50 ml of aloe vera gel

Application
Offer the remedy to the animal. Apply to the affected areas 2 x daily. As the condition begins to clear, apply 1 x daily or as needed. Most of the redness should have disappeared after a couple of days. Skin scrapes taken by the vet have been seen to be clear within a week after the application of the above oils.

Fleas / mites / midges

10 g powdered clay or chalk
10 drops tea tree
1-3 drops neem oil
Place in a bag and shake well.

Application
Offer the remedy to the animal. Apply to the coat, especially under the armpits, back of the neck and top of the tail. Leave on for 1 hour and then comb through with a flea comb. Do this every three days for two weeks.

Also offer oils to support the immune system.

Caution: some animals have an adverse reaction to tea tree oil so it is important to offer it to the animal before application.

Daisy, a cat with fleas
Tamara Roberts

I combed Daisy with a flea comb and placed three fleas in individual jars. I put one drop of tea tree oil in one of the jars and within seconds the flea was immobilised. In the other jar I put one drop of citronella and noted no change to the fleas behaviour. In the third jar I put a drop of neem oil and observed the flea hopping around frantically. I left the jars for forty minutes; on my return the tea tree flea was still immobilised and presumed dead, the citronella flea was busy climbing around the sides of the jar avoiding the citronella, and the neem flea was still frantically hopping around.

In response to the above experiment I combined tea tree, neem oil and powdered chalk, in hope to achieve a flea killer and deterrent. I mixed one drop of neem and one drop of tea tree to 10g of powdered chalk. I rubbed this into Daisy's coat, paying particular attention to the back of her neck, base of her tail and armpits. Thirty minutes later I flea combed her and removed seven dead fleas. That evening Daisy was more restful. I repeated the treatment every three days for two weeks (to stop the flea cycle), even though only the first session collected fleas in the flea comb.

Dying

Allowing animals into our lives very often means that we will have to face their physical death, something for which most of us are never fully prepared.

Frankincense, spikenard and rose have been used for thousands of years in the embalming of bodies and for burial rituals, in the belief that they clear the spirit in preparation for the next life. You may find that animals will often select these oils at this time.

Essential oils can really help to comfort an animal at this time, and also the owner. Oils such as frankincense, spikenard and rose help take fears away and allow the animal to 'let go' in peace clearing their way for their next journey.

Application

Add 5 drops of the selected oil to a bowl (approximately 200ml) of warm water. Dip your hands into it, then gently stroke in a long slow motion over the animals body. Inhalation alone may be preferred.

working with different species equine, canine, feline

The principals of Animal Aromatics remain the same for any species. Whether you are using essential oils with horses, dogs, cats or more exotic animals, try and learn how the individual species behave and medicate themselves in the wild, as I have outlined in this section. This will give you a better idea of how to work with them.

Given the choice, animals will usually select plants and their extracts from plant families similar to those that are indigenous to their habitat. For example, horses flown over from Bahrain were mainly interested in oils that grew in their home region such as rose, frankincense, jasmine and sandalwood. Working with a species you are unfamiliar with can be daunting at first. A little research and close observation will be of great help to you. Be patient, use your intuition and knowledge and you will get results.

If in doubt call the vet for any condition, no matter how minor it appears

Equine (and most herbivores)

Herbivores eat plants containing essential oils and so have metabolic pathways that enable them to break down most essential oils. In the wild they will naturally treat themselves orally. However aromatics are also applied to the skin to treat a variety of isolated conditions, usually by putting the appropriate oils into an aloe vera gel base. For example, peppermint would be put in a gel to numb areas causing itching and cool the skin; German chamomile and yarrow are used to help with inflammatory responses, as well as for their cooling effects, garlic is applied to deter mites and help prevent secondary infections and Dead Sea mineral mud to protect and heal the skin further. Mud is commonly applied in the wild for many afflictions as well as to deter biting insects.

Remedies frequently selected by horses

All the essential oils in this book are appropriate to offer horses, however the most commonly selected are:

Essential oils and plant extracts
Angelica root
Bergamot
Carrot seed
Cederwood
Chamomile Roman
Chamomile German
Frankincense
Garlic
Jasmine
Juniperberry
Linden blossom
Lotus pink
Neroli
Peppermint
Rose otto / rose absolute
Sandalwood
Sea buckthorn
Seaweed
Valerian
Vanilla
Vetiver
Violet leaf
Yarrow
Ylang ylang

Macerated oils
Arnica
Comfrey
Marigold
St John's wort

Fixed oils
Safflower (thistle)
Sunflower
Olive

Other remedies
Clay
Cornflower water
Dead Sea mineral mud
Devil's claw tubers
Dried rosehips
Licorice root

Number remedies generally selected
3-7 essential oils
1-3 macerated
Dried remedies such as devil's claw, rosehips and
Possibly cornflower water

Remedies for common problems

Wounds

Yarrow

Use on broken skin and in conditions where pus exudes from the wound. I would recommend that everyone has this oil in their possession, if for nothing else, than the treatment of wounds; in my opinion yarrow evolved for such afflictions, its ability to heal wounds is truly amazing. Yarrow is a powerful anti-inflammatory that helps to reduce swelling, sooth inflamed tissues and neutralise excess heat and pain, while providing an environment where it is difficult for bacteria to grow. Yarrow also helps to release the trauma associated with the wound, so could be used as a rescue remedy.

Undiluted on open wounds

Drop onto the wound until the area stains blue, the amount needed will be absorbed, once the skin stains blue, the body has had enough. For larger areas add yarrow to an aloe vera gel.

Carrot seed

Controls excessive bleeding (especially when taken orally). It is indicated for internal cell damage. Offer orally.

Seaweed: Protects and seals the wound, draws out impurities and prevents the invasion of foreign bodies. Seaweed contains iodine, an antiseptic sulphur, noted for its blood purifying and anti-bacterial action; magnesium for nerve function and zinc, renowned for its wound-healing and immune stimulating properties. Use undiluted or in aloe gel.

Dead Sea mineral mud

Flies are particularly attracted to wounds. Dead Sea mineral mud is a useful deterrent as well as having healing properties of its own. It is not unusual for elephants to use mud in the wild to help heal wounds as well as to protect the skin from insects.

Clay

Dry clay sprinkled onto an oozing wound, will help to dry it and protect it from infection.

Clay can also be made into a paste by adding water, this would be applied to help draw out impurities.

German chamomile

Indicated for skin repair and proud flesh. Use undiluted or in an aloe gel.

Sea buckthorn or lavender

Enhances the formation of cell tissue. It improves granulation. Use undiluted topically and offer orally.

First aid wound gel

50ml aloe gel
6 drops yarrow
1ml (20/30 drops) seaweed

Offer arnica and rose for shock

> **Remedies for the tack room**
> Arnica macerated oil
> Comfrey macerated oil
> Devils claw tubers (keep in air tight container)
> Dried rosehips
> Yarrow essential oil

Arthritis, joint / ligament problems and inflammation

Including ringbone, navicular and splints

Usually taken orally or inhaled

Arnica	bruising / shock
Carrot seed	cell repair
Comfrey	inflammation, pulled muscles, tendons and ligaments
Chalk	joint / bone degeneration disorders / splints
Devil's claw	analgesic / anti-inflammatory
Garlic	thins the blood - navicular / ringbone / laminitis
Lime / juniper	splints
Peppermint	stimulates circulation (useful while on box rest) / analgesic
Seaweed	lack of movement / repair
Yarrow / German chamomile	anti-inflammatory

Use where there is heat or swelling: offer orally / make into a gel:

Immortelle	bruising, cell regenerating
Peppermint	anti-inflammatory: deep heat-ice pack effect
Valerian	deep muscle relaxant
Wintergreen	analgesic, deep heat, warming / healing
Yarrow	tissue inflammation

Add a total of 25-50 drops of essential oil to 150 ml of gel, depending on the severity of the condition. Apply to the affected area 1-2 x daily or as needed. Reduce the frequency of the application as the horse indicates.

Pain relief / anti-inflammatory gel

Peppermint	20 - 40 drops
Wintergreen (horses)	10 -20 drops
Yarrow	2 - 4 drops

Blend into 150 ml gel. Add more drops or use less gel if a stronger application is required. Apply to the affected area 1-2 x daily or as needed. Reduce the frequency of the application as the horse indicates. Allow the horse to lick gels off the hand if it chooses to do so.

Tumours / Sarcoids / Warts

The treatment of sarcoids and tumours is not always straightforward. As with most conditions the behavioural element needs to be addressed as well as the symptoms. Oils to support the liver and kidneys, the primary organs for cleansing the body and oils for the immune system should also be considered. I have found that horses with tumours and sarcoids will usually include oils that are photo-reactive in their selection.

Photo- reactive oils that are often selected
Angelica root - (not seed)
Bergamot
St John's wort

Seaweed extract and carrot seed essential oil, are also frequently selected. They are not photo-reactive but help support the liver.

Offer for inhalation and orally. Topically they can be applied in an aloe gel, beeswax, clay or mud. Clay and Dead Sea mineral mud are generally used on dry nodular sarcoids, whereas gels or beeswax are used on other types. If the sarcoid is bloody it is best not to apply anything topically.

Gel is used for rapid absorption
Clay is used to protect or dry the sarcoid / wart, to help it shrivel up and drop off.

Apply 1-2 x daily or as needed. Sarcoids have been known to drop off within days of application, while others have taken months, even a year with the animal selecting oils intermittently until the scarcoid or wart has dropped off or reabsorbed into the body, after a while they will loose interest in their remedies. If the sarcoids drops off over night it may cause the area to bleed slightly, however this occurence is more unusual.

Laminitis

Laminitis is not fully understood, but one of the main contributory factors lies with the consumption of fast growing spring and late summer grass. In both cases its rapid growth results in a low mineral content and high carbohydrate levels. Concussion is another common cause, as well as toxins in the blood.

The horses blood pressure is prone to rise, and there is a reduced blood flow to the capillary beds that supply the sensitive laminae in the hoof. Blood clots can sometimes form, further impairing circulation. In almost every laminitic case, seaweed extract or absolute is selected, (abundant minerals / nutrients) as well as German chamomile; for severe cases great mugwort (both are antihistemic / anti-inflammatory) and neroli for separation which is probably why ponies suffer more frequently. Noticeable results can usually be seen within days of the horse taking selected oils, even with horses that have not been expected to recover.

Remedies to offer (inhalation and oral)

Arnica	bruising/anti-inflammatory
Devil's claw	pain/anti-inflammatory
Chamomile German	anti-histaminic
great mugwort	anti-histaminic (strong)
Neroli	separation
Rose	trauma
Seaweed	balances nutrients/detox
St John's wort	depression/nerve damage

Also offer flouve, garlic, carrot seed, peppermint

Pain relieving gel
20 drops peppermint
20 drops wintergreen
Add to 50 ml aloe vera gel

Application: Offer the remedy to the horse, apply to the coronet band as needed.

Sweet itch

Sweet itch is believed to be an allergic reaction to the saliva of the Culicoides midge. The reaction causes severe irritation, itching and raw patches, mainly on the poll, mane, trunk and base of the tail. The rubbing of these areas can cause further damage to the skin and infection can occur. All horses can be affected by this allergy, but ponies, cobs and Icelandic breeds seem to suffer more frequently.

Lavender	15 drops - healing to the skin
Neem oil	2 ml - deters midges
Peppermint	30 drops - numbs the itch
German chamomile	6 drops - anti-histaminic
Roman chamomile	7 drops - skin /anxiety
Yarrow	5 drops - healing / inflammation
Garlic	7-8 drops - secondary infection

Application

Add to 150ml aloe vera gel. If the horse indicates that any oil is needed individually either for inhalation or for oral use, also make up separate bottles. Apply 1-2 x daily, or as needed.

Offer when the first signs of itching appear. In severe cases add more German chamomile and yarrow, which will help draw out the heat, itch and pain as well as being healing to the tissues. Extra peppermint could also be applied to help control the itch whilst warding off the midges.

Signs of improvement should be seen within 24 hours. Also offer oils to match the animal's temperament. Allow the horse to lick the gel if chosen. It is not unusual for horses in the wild to roll in mud to protect themselves from fly bites and midges. I have found that applying Dead Sea mineral mud after the applying the gel really helps deter the midges, while protecting and healing affected skin.

Note: Recently I have found that horses are selecting orange and blood orange essential oil when they are suffering from sweet itch, sometimes taking up to 20 mls a day at a 50% dilution. These horses also seem to enjoy fresh whole oranges. On one occasion when the horse was denied his daily essential oil of orange, due to the owner going on holiday, the sweet itch manifested itself instantly. When she returned two weeks later most of the mane had been lost. The horse resumed to taking the remedies again with relish for a further two weeks; then went on to having just the gel and Dead Sea mineral mud applied. The condition once again became under control with hair growing back.

Base oils may exacerbate the condition.

Colic

Colic includes a variety of conditions in which the horse suffers abdominal pain. If the horse exhibits even mild abdominal discomfort, the vet should be called. While waiting for the vet offer the remedies below, discomfort can sometimes be relieved immediately.

Spasmodic colic	Roman / German chamomile
Impactions	peppermint
Gastric	peppermint / seaweed / fennel
Tympanitic (unsuitable food)	seaweed / peppermint / fennel
Stress related	Roman / German chamomile
Worm damage	Carrot seed

In many cases a 50% dilution is needed. Allow the horse to take as much as required. Refer to case study in the dilution section of this book.

Mud fever

The *Dermatophilus congolensis* bacterium is mainly found in cattle, sheep, goats and horses. Horses are the most commonly effected, the condition is rarely seen in cats and dogs. The bacteria found in the soil, usually make their way through wet skin but can enter through injuries and are also transmitted by ticks and biting flies. Factors such as skin pigmentation, malnutrition, stress and heredity have also been reported to play an important part in the spread of the condition in susceptible animals. In severe cases the skin becomes very sore and inflamed, with a serum exudate, that causes matted hair.

In the study on *Dermotophilus congolensis* (refer to profiles on garlic) garlic was seen to completely inhibit the growth of the bacteria. Remedies to support the constitution of the animal need to be taken into consideration, in order to prevent further outbreaks. It is interesting to note that mud fever has been successfully treated with thyme and/or lavender; yet in laboratory conditions garlic was the only oil out of these three, that showed complete inhibition of the bacteria. This clearly demonstrates to me that essential oils should be used and understood holistically.

Garlic / red thyme / bay laurel	7 drops
Roman chamomile	7 drops
Yarrow	4 drops
German chamomile	4 - 6 drops
Add to 150ml aloe gel.	

Severe cases may need bitter almond essential oil (the hydrocyanic will have been removed). Roman chamomile is normally selected as an oral remedy.

Application

Offer the remedy to the horse. Apply undiluted 1-2 x daily or as needed. There is no need to remove scabs. If no improvement is seen within a week seek, professional advice. Allow your horse to lick the gel from the hand.

If the mud fever is so severe that large cracks appear in the skin, make up a loose beeswax remedy using a selected macerated or fixed oil and add seaweed and German chamomile. Apply to the cracks. This will act as a barrier and provide rapid healing to the area.

Rain scald

The same bacterium as in mud fever, *Dermatophilus congolensis*, causes rain scald. Treat in a similar way, if secondary infection is present, a thick layer of pus will be found under the scabs. In this case you may need to add more garlic, either way - let your vet know.

Thrush

Ensure that the animal is kept in clean dry conditions and ask the farrier or bare foot specialist to trim any dead tissue. Brush tea tree, bay laurel or manuka onto the foot 1-2 x daily or as needed. Offer seaweed extract and rosehips orally to help boost the immune system.

Poor circulation to the feet can be a contributing cause of thrush, so it may also help to offer circulation stimulants, such as peppermint.

Hoof moisturiser

The hoof is modified skin. The wall, sole, frog and periople are derived from the epidermis. Some horses have a thin hoof wall with slow growth, the wall may also crack and become brittle. Sand cracks and grass cracks can also be a problem. In addition to good management, i.e having the feet regularly trimmed and not allowing the horn to become excessively dry, offer carrot seed essential oil, which contains carotol that stimulates the regeneration of cells. The macerated carrot base oil contains carotene which converts to vitamin A, responsible for keeping coat, gums and teeth healthy. Applied together to the hoof and offered orally, they work miraculously to restore healthy hooves.

It is now commonly thought that hoof oil keeps the moisture out rather than in. Hooves are more susceptible to dry out and crack when the weather is dry. The best thing would be to walk them through a stream twice a day - but not very workable!

Carrot seed   1 ml
Garlic   5 drops

Add to 50ml aloe vera gel (let down with a little water to make it a firm but not too sticky consistency)

Also offer orally
Rosehips
Rosemary
Sea buckthorn
Seaweed extract

Application
Offer and apply as needed.

Fly repellent

I have noticed that after horses have been treated with aromatics, either orally or by inhalation, the flies that had previously hung around them often disappear. This could be because flies tend to gravitate to stagnant blood or energy.

It is interesting to observe the area of the body to which the flies gravitate. For some horses it will be the head, others the stomach or eyes and so on. If flies collect around the stomach a depleted energy in the stomach meridian could be indicated. If they are around the eyes, which in Chinese medicine are connected to the liver, offer oils to support the liver and so on.

However, horses ridden down country lanes and past bushes will be irritated by flies regardless, in this case apply the general fly gel.

General fly gel
Add 30 drops peppermint to 1-2ml neem oil. Most horses do not have a problem with peppermint and it is not photo-reactive like essential oils used in many commercial sprays.

As a wipe
Add to 150ml aloe gel and shake well. Using a cloth, wipe in the direction of the coat, avoiding the eyes. Very often horses will want to take this orally - that is fine if they choose to do so. Watery mud around the face is always a good choice, but cosmetically not an owner's first choice!

As a spray
Add to 250ml of very watery aloe gel. Shake well and spray. Avoid the eyes.

Splints

A splint is a bony enlargement of the splint bone. In young horses it is subject to strain and tear, causing bleeding and proliferation of fibrous tissue, resulting in inflammation and the production of new bone. Offer the following: Remedies marked with* can be added to a gel.

Yarrow*	anti-inflammatory
German chamomile*	anti-inflammatory
Carrot seed	repair
Chalk	promotes healthy bones
Lime	breaks down debris
Garlic	blood thinning
Peppermint*	cooling / analgesic
Wintergreen*	anti-inflammatory/ analgesic
Arnica	anti-inflammatory/trauma
Devil's claw	anti-inflammatory/ analgesic

Offer and apply as needed.

Sun screen

Lavender	7-10 drops
Peppermint	5-7 drops

Add to 50ml aloe vera gel, or add to clay mixed with aloe vera gel or dead sea mud. The clay and mud help offer added protection but make sure it does not become too drying as this would be uncomfortable for the horse.

Fruits and vegetables containing beta-carotenes and flavonoids, offer protection from the sun's rays to the skin, so it would possibly be beneficial to also offer remedies such as rosehips, sea buckthorn and carrot macerate. Sometimes horses will select bergamot which appears to rebalance pigmentation, but can cause a photo-sensitive reaction when it is not needed.

Travelling

The warm humid air given off from the animal's body and breath provides an ideal breeding ground for bacteria whilst travelling by horsebox. Oils to suit such conditions are those that are volatile and antiseptic, such as bergamot and garlic, bergamot being a first choice for most people! These oils emit vapours that provide a hostile environment for bacteria. Bergamot is uplifting oil that can also help counteract the stress of travelling and is popular with most animals.

Antiseptic spray

Garlic	5-7 drops
Bergamot	10-20 drops

Add either, garlic, bergamot or both to an aloe vera gel and let down with enough water to make into a spray.

Application

Offer the remedy to the horse. Spray onto the sides of the trailer / box or wipe along the animal's neck in the direction of the coat.

Horse box / trailer problems

Problems with boxing are common and can prove to be very distressing for both the horse and the people involved. Essential oils can be offered straight away, before any travelling takes place as the problem lays dormant within the horse, only manifesting itself at the time it is boxed. Rose otto is a useful oil to have at hand if remedies have not been offered prior to travel.

Oils to offer (for inhalation and orally)

Clary sage
Frankincense
Jasmine
Rose otto
Valerian
Vetiver
Violet leaf

When the horse no longer requires the remedies, re-offer them minutes before boxing, and again during boxing.

Travel rub

Travelling frequently causes muscular pain, since the animals have to constantly brace their legs in very unnatural positions for long periods of time, with no warning as to braking, corners and bouncing on uneven road surfaces. The muscles mainly involved are the shoulders, back, loins, quarters and upper legs, which when strained may release lactic acid that can cause pain and possible muscle damage. Horses that then have to work on arrival at their destination will not perform as fluently if the muscles are strained or tight.

Invigorating rub

Peppermint   20 drops (stimulates circulation)
Juniper berry   20 drops (dispels lactic acid)
Mix into 150ml loose gel.

Application
Offer the remedy to the horse. Use as needed.

Rub down

Peppermint   20 drops (stimulant)
Juniper   10 drops (dispels lactic acid)
Lavender   15 drops (muscle relaxant)
Marjoram sweet 6 drops (muscle relaxant)

Mix into 150 ml loose gel.

Application
Offer the remedy to the horse. Use as needed.

NOTE: Essential oils have not been tested for their legal use with competition horses, they therefore should be regarded as medicines.

Case studies: equine

Vaccine reaction
Sharon King 2005

The morning after the vaccination Kappella was found standing in her field unable to walk, however, with some encouragement she was able to hobble from her field to the stable, she was so lame that her back legs appeared to be crossing over one another; she also appeared very stiff and in a lot of pain. The vet was called immediately. He noticed a small lump on her neck at the site of the injection and suspected an adverse reaction to the vaccine, so Kappella was given a pain killing injection and phenybutazone. Later that day the small lump had become a massive swelling covering one side of her neck. The vet returned diagnosed a haematoma (an accumulation of blood within the tissues), and suggested massage and more phenybutazone. Kappella couldn't stand her neck to be touched so massage was out of the question. She was also unable to lower her head to graze. The next day the swelling was even worse and Kappella was very depressed. The vet was called yet again. He thought there may now be an abscess and advised continuing with phenybutazone. Two days later there was no improvement, Kappella continued to look depressed and appeared to be in considerable pain. At this point his owner was advised to buy an over the counter arnica cream but this did not seem to help. Three days after the injection, her owner asked if I could help Kappella with essential oils and I made up the following remedies:

When I arrived Kappella was lying down in her stable; she got up very slowly and stood facing the wall which was very unlike her. She seemed very depressed. Kappella inhaled both yarrow and carrot seed with one nostril but didn't want more. I then tried the yarrow gel that I had made up, massaging it into her neck using gentle downward strokes, which she tolerated. After this she was much more interested in the yarrow and the carrot seed, so I applied more yarrow and added some carrot seed to her neck gel. The difference from the first application to the second was amazing. Kappella started to lean into my downward strokes and after 5 minutes I had to brace myself on the stable wall to apply the amount of pressure she was asking for. I continued massaging and it seemed that with each stroke the swelling was reducing. After 30 minutes all that remained were two small lumps at the base of her neck. When I left the stable she carried on massaging the area herself, rubbing against the stable door. The pain had obviously gone. Later that day Kappella wanted more yarrow on her neck but didn't want any the following day. She seemed a lot happier in herself and was almost back to normal so I didn't feel it was necessary to give her phenybutazone that night. However, she was still having difficulty lowering her head.

When the vet called by the next day he was very keen to know how the swelling had reduced so quickly. I then decided to offer peppermint (for pain, bruising, heat and nerve damage), and immortelle (for bruising and scar tissue). Kappella turned away from immortelle but loved peppermint. She inhaled it with both nostrils and licked about six drops from my hand with the underside of her tongue. She also allowed me to stroke some onto her neck, but only where there was bruising. I added 10 drops of peppermint to 10ml of water and left the remedy with her owner to continue the treatment.

When I visited Kapella four days later she still couldn't reach the ground to graze so I offered the following oils: wintergreen, juniper berry and yarrow and peppermint.

Kapella inhaled them all, though peppermint seemed to be her favourite. I added 10 drops of wintergreen, 5 drops of yarrow, 15 drops of peppermint and 5 drops of juniper to 150ml of aloe vera gel. I applied the remedy to her neck and 20 minutes later she was eating her hay from the ground! Her owner was delighted. Kappella was the first animal I had treated with essential oils and the whole experience was amazing.

Remedies selected by Kappella
Oral
Yarrow 8 drops in 10ml base oil (to reduce bleeding, swelling, heat, pain and help with the trauma). Carrot seed 8 drops in 10ml of water (to stop the bleeding and for cell repair).

In aloe vera gel: topical
Yarrow 10 drops in 60ml of aloe vera gel and water, for topical application.

A horse with a sarcoid
Caroline Ingraham 2006

Shadow is an 8 year old bay pure bred Arab. We have had him for three years. He is a very sensitive, reactive type but quite bold and curious. In the past he has had unexplained hard skin nodules down one flank which did not respond to the vets topical treatment but disappeared when he stopped being shod and fed molasses. When I first noticed the sarcoid it was a grey spherical lump about the size of a bean. It was red and raw around the edges. It is situated at the inside top of his right fore, by the armpit. I am not aware of any trauma to the area. He didn't seem bothered by it but when I returned from holiday it seemed to have grown a lump on top of the original lump. It is hard to say how long it had been there before I noticed it as it is a hidden place. Also Shadow's rider has not had as much time for him since she started her A' levels. He is a very friendly one-person horse so I am sure that he is feeling sad about this.

Offered in the evening
Cornflower water: opens up to healing
Melissa (antiviral)
Angelica root (photo-reactive)
Neroli (loss/ separation)
Roman chamomile (skin / anxiety problems)

Offered in the morning
Arnica
Carrot seed
Seaweed
Peppermint
Garlic

Topical, applied to the sarcoid
Dead Sea mud with several drops of angelica root and melissa added, if he does not want it applied he will walk away.

Update: Strange (& interesting) developments today. When I went to call the horses from the field for their breakfast (and oils), Merlin came down but there was no sign of Shadow, who normally races Merlin to the gate. I put Merlin in and went to look for Shadow and found him lying down in a sunny spot at the top of the field (this is pretty unusual).

He is very keen on the arnica and seaweed, also carrot seed and peppermint to a lesser extent. In the evening, when I called them in, again Merlin came and Shadow didn't. It was pitch dark and I didn't fancy looking for him but luckily he came after I'd taken Merlin in and gone back and called a few times. He didn't seem interested in his oils, so I tried them all again and he just wasn't interested. I waited and eventually tried again after a few minutes and then he was interested in the cornflower and licked some of that, but not the others (melissa, angelica, neroli, chamomile). He was just about interested enough in the mud for me to apply it.

Update
On the whole Shadow seems generally calmer, the lump does appear better. I am sure it has shrunk. He has lost interest in all but a few oils now - nearly all the 'emotional' ones are getting no response - even the cornflower, which he was very interested in before, only gets a passing sniff. He is still very interested in: arnica macerate, carrot seed, seaweed, peppermint (not as much as he was, and the first three noticeably more than the last one). Shadow continued to take seaweed intermittently, for four months until it was noticed that just a slight hard patch remained where the sarcoid was. He continues to be well.

Authors note
On two occasions I have experienced sarcoids falling off over night. The first was with a horse that took St John's wort essential oil orally with nothing applied topically, in the morning the sarcoids had come off leaving a hole where it had been and the leg slightly stained with a trickle of blood. We packed the hole with clay and seaweed - this healed remarkably quickly. The smaller sarcoid on the other side of the body was reabsorbed a couple of days later.

The second occasion was reported back from a student who had applied bergamot topically in aloe vera gel to a cluster of warts - and offered carrot seed and seaweed, which was taken orally. The warts fell off over night.

Horse with Sarcoids
Dawn Featherstone 2006

I have been offering remedies to a horse with sarcoids since 8th February. In brief the horse was showing signs of sarcoids on the inside / upper thigh area (off hind leg) at the beginning of the year - He initially had bergamot applied in a gel, which he only allowed to be applied for 2 days. Orally he took, carrot Seed, seaweed extract, rosehips, marigold macerate, St John's wort, sea buckthorn, yarrow - and then about a month later he started to take lemon. Over the course of several months the sarcoids have been 'growing' (I think to date that at least 15 sarcoids have appeared and disappeared) - they go through a process of 'ballooning up', weeping and sometimes bleeding then disappearing. It has been quite amazing to see the process, as when the sarcoids are going through what I call their 'explosive state' he stops taking all of the oils - then once they have settled down again he will take all his remedies - as if restarting and clearing for the next 'batch'.

Behavioural problems
Sara De Vries 2004

Billy is a gorgeous little pony, he is in good condition and fit. Billy is very different with the little girl that rode him over the past few years than he was with anyone else. With her he was calm and well behaved, but he was very nervous with other people, so much so that sometimes he would rear, refuse to load and fall back on the lead rope. It was as if he was two different ponies.

Billy had previously been very cruelly treated, consequently he has gone from home to home. Unfortunately, the little girl that he bonded with grew out of him and her parents purchased her a new pony, fortunately her new pony is at the same yard as Billy, so he will still see and hear her. Another girl will start to ride him, although they are going to do this very gradually. I have suggested that the new girl offers him neroli.

When I offered plant remedies to Billy he selected cornflower water, arnica macerated oil, linden blossom, valerian, vetiver and violet leaf. The oils elicited a strong to medium interest for three weeks, however his preference was to violet leaf, of which he took 25 mls (diluted in base oil) in the first 10 days, and continued to show a strong interest. When I visited the yard about one and half weeks after Billy began his remedies he appeared more confident. One of the girls came up to me and said that he had been really good over the past few days. I asked if she thought it was due to the oils and she replied 'oh I don't know about that'. It was nice that someone saw a change without preconceived ideas. The little girl who now owns him also has seen a lot of changes in him. She felt that he was no longer spooky or nervous of things that really worried him before, that he became easier to handle and was better when ridden. I actually saw him in a show about three weeks into the case study. He was in a jumping class, he was the smallest there, and he bombed around the course as if confidence was going to explode out of him. He won the first round and then the jump off, finishing first and earning a trophy. I felt myself filling with tears, thinking about what people had once done to him and seeing how far this gorgeous little boy had come. That evening when I visited the yard to pick up the reaction sheet, I went to his stable and over he came for a fuss, giving a little neigh. He would never have done that before - what more of a perfect ending could I have asked for.

The little girl's mum also has a horse at the yard and she has always been a complete non believer in anything alternative. Since seeing the dramatic results in Billy she has now become fascinated and asked if I could work with her horse.

Pure Breed Arab: Run down
Elizabeth Soames 2006

Jo is an honest horse and will try to work well for you however he is feeling. He is fed, Hi-Fi original chaff, Pink powders, Cortiflex powders, ad-lib hay and grass turn out. He moved to the yard about five years ago, having previously been out on loan where his rider had started to struggle with him. His care had been reduced and he was like a wound up spring to ride, so therefore never got ridden. His present owner took him back and put him in the riding school where he is now, as a working livery. Since his arrival I took Jo on the loan scheme where I hack and have lessons. Jo has a fear of mares as he was attacked by one when he was a year old, he now lives next to a very highly strung mare.

The first signs of concern was when Jo, aged seventeen years, became low on energy with his coat looking dull. He began to lose weight so he was given dietary supplements (he also had a worm count done), this offered some improvement to his condition. Then out of the blue he then started to shut his eyes whilst being ridden in the school. At this point he was stabled. He began to stare into space, seemingly concentrating on standing up - I wondered if he was feeling dizzy? He went completely off his food and had very pale mucous membranes.

Treatment

When Jo was stabled, I offered him plant oils and extracts. He was so shut down, but after a little while he turned and put his head out and watched, as I tested his hair using kinesiology, to see what was needed. I found a lack of energy on both sides of his liver, stomach and pancreas. The oils that he selected were rose absolute, wild carrot seed, yarrow, lemon and spirulina. As I was selecting the oils, Jo got more and more interested in them and started to push me, trying to get at them.

I offered Jo the oils individually while he was loose in the stable so that he could get away from the aroma if he chose to. I started with rose, he took long smells using both nostrils, and he then licked and tried to snatch the bottle, so I put some into the palm of my hand where he licked it up using both sides of his tongue.

Next I offered him the wild carrot seed, he didn't even appear to smell the bottle but went straight to lick and snatch at it so I put some in my hand and again he licked, nibbling at my hand for more. He took quite a lot of this oil and seemed quite desperate for it.

Next I offered him yarrow. He smelt the yarrow using each nostril in turn and then tried to lick the bottle. I gave him some on my hand which he licked, he then did the flehmen response and then came back for more rubbing his lips into my hand and covering his nostrils in it before licking.

Finally I offered him the lemon, he smelt the oil with both nostrils and once again tried to snatch the bottle. I offered it to him on the palm of my hand and he licked it up using both sides of his tongue, he wanted to take quite a lot of this oil.

I placed the spirulina into a clean feed bowl and mixed it with a little water and offered it to Jo. He put his lips into it and wiggled them about covering his whole mouth area, he then did the flehmen reaction while covering the stable in spirulina - but he seemed to enjoy it.

Within a few minutes of Jo taking the oils he brightened up and lost the dazed look he had earlier, he then turned and started to slowly eat his hay, taking more interest in his surroundings again, whinnying as if to say thank you. Jo took all the oils both orally and by inhaled every day for a week, snatching at the bottles in desperation every time they were brought out. In the first week when his need for them was so strong, he would leave food to take them.

By the end of the first week he had a good pink colour back in his mucous membranes, his energy level had increased with his appetite and his coat had started to improve. He only took the spirulina for the first two days before losing interest, but it had probably given him the required boost for him to start the healing process.

During the second week the urgency for the remedies had gone from Jo and he started to lose interest in the rose absolute and carrot seed, which he mainly inhaled. He was still taking the yarrow and lemon orally reduced to a couple of drops of each at a time. By the beginning of the third week he had lost interest in most of the oils.

Physical and Behavioural Changes
Within a few minutes of Jo having his oils he started to look brighter and began to eat again. The main change was in his eyes, he looked like he was back with us instead of shut down or dazed.

By the next day Jo was calling as soon as I stepped on to the yard and was waiting at the door of the stable for me. As soon as I went to the cupboard for his oils he would become very pushy and try to get in with me, I had to guard the oils to stop him swallowing the bottles! As he began to feel better he became calmer and would whinny gently, wanting cuddles, pushing his head into my arms. He would then go and eat heartily instead of picking at his food.

By the end of the first week had had a good pink colour back in his mucous membranes, his energy level had increased along with his appetite and his coat had started to improve, his character had come back and his eyes no longer looked distant. He strode out with purpose again and seemed to be more tolerant of mares, letting them come slightly closer. His whole body condition continues to improve and his weight is increasing. He no longer trips when he is ridden either. I feel the oils he selected helped to boost his immune system and fight off illness. He also selected oils to help him to cope better with the mare that lived next door to him, this had an overall calming effect on his behaviour.

Jo is back to his springy self and has re-found the lust for life, but with it he is more centred and things don't seem to scare him as much; he spooks and jumps less too. He seems happier and more secure in himself. I may still have no brakes when we are on the fields, but he is much less likely to do anything daft like he did before.

A horse with leg wounds
Karen Douglas 2004

One evening Max and I were working in the sand school. After he finished working I took his tack off him to let him have a roll. He lay down quite near to the fence, rubbed his neck and his side in the sand then, unfortunately, decided to roll over appearing to have forgotten how close to the fence he was. He caught his leg on the second rail of the fence and in his anxiety about being caught, began to thrash his leg, scraping it repeatedly against the fencing pulling a heavy metal spreader down. He freed himself and got up but hobbled away on three legs.

Within seconds I could see a large haematoma forming on the inside of his thigh and there were a number of cuts, all of which were bleeding. Fortunately, after a while he seemed happy to put his weight on the injured leg so I walked him up the yard and called the vet.

While I waited for the vet to arrive, I offered Max oils that I felt were going to be helpful in the very early stages of the trauma - rose, arnica macerated oil, yarrow, comfrey and carrot seed.

Max wanted to lick lots of arnica and yarrow. He sniffed the rose but was not interested in licking it. The vet arrived within 20 minutes of the accident, by which time some of the haematoma had already started to go down. He examined Max, found nothing to be broken and said the wounds were not suitable for stitching. He offered to give Max antibiotic and anti-inflammatory drugs as a precaution. I explained that I wanted to use the oils and he was agreeable to this, suggesting that cold hosing the leg would also help reduce any swelling.

After the vet had gone I offered Max more arnica and yarrow, both of which he wanted to lick. I then cold hosed his leg and applied neat yarrow to the wounds.

Max was also interested in taking carrot seed, dandelion, clivers and nettle. I then offered seaweed, tea tree, thyme and calendula but he was not interested in these.

Max has a 24 hour turn out, so the vet thought that it was wise to continue this regime as he felt box rest would add to the swelling. Max grazed with his companions but did not walk as far as he normally would.

The following morning there was extensive swelling and inflammation around the hock. The swelling had also tracked down to the fetlock, although this was less swollen. The wounds themselves looked very good, clean, no bleeding. Where there was sufficient yarrow the tissues remained stained blue, where more yarrow was needed the wounds appeared red. Max continued to want to lick arnica, yarrow and carrot seed and he also wanted to eat dandelion root, clivers and nettle.

Within 48 hours Max was no longer selecting arnica macerated oil and the swelling had reduced, he now wanted comfrey. He continued to want yarrow and carrot seed orally. He no longer wanted nettle but continued to select dandelion. I also applied more yarrow to the wounds. Max selected sweet marjoram (stiffness) and peppermint, (stimulates circulation, nerve function and anti-inflammatory), both of which he took orally. The wounds continued to make excellent progress and the stiffness in his leg became less noticeable. Within 72 hours of the accident the swelling had almost disappeared and Max was fully mobile. He continued to select comfrey, yarrow, carrot seed and peppermint orally and just inhaled the sweet marjoram. After a while he started to want German chamomile, taking it orally. Four days after the accident Max trotted and cantered over the field with no apparent stiffness. The swelling to the hock and fetlock was minimal, he continued to select comfrey, yarrow, carrot seed and German chamomile.

Summery of progress

Max gradually stopped taking the oils, and became interested only in rosehip shells which he took for five days. The wounds had granulated on two areas and there had been signs of proud flesh developing, I offered lavender, which Max showed a positive response to, so I put it neat on the areas that had granulated.

Max was sound and able to hack out within a week. The wounds remained infection free and have healed without leaving any scarring or white hair areas.

A horse with laminitis
Sharon Stewart 2004

Connie is an eight year old grey Highland mare, who, several years ago had a bout of laminitis. Again she became severely lame with suspected laminitis. The vet prescribed phenylbutazone and ACP (a tranquilliser which dilates blood vessels and helps improve blood flow to the foot) to relieve pain and calm her. The usual routine of restricted grazing and padding the feet followed. Connie selected rose otto, seaweed, peppermint and carrot seed from the oils I offered, which she took orally. I also left carrot macerate oil and some devil's claw tubers.

Connie's owner phoned later that evening to say that she had perked up no end and was looking a lot less sad. Her owner then had to go away for a couple of days, but on her return called me up to ask how quickly the oils would take effect. My immediate thought was that Connie was no better, but on the contrary, the owner had been amazed to find a sound, gleaming, healthy looking horse that four days previously had been very lame and depressed with laminitis.

Note: Very often laminitic ponies also select arnica, German chamomile and neroli.

Sore feet
Viv Williams 2006

Gino is a 15 year old Hanoverian gelding that competes at dressage level. He is fed hard feed and hay twice a day with just hay at lunch time and is ridden or lunged 6 days a week with turnout as well. He can only work on soft surfaces so can't be hacked on roads or even hard tracks due to his highly sensitive feet. His owner has tried various types of shoes and he has been checked by the vet. He does not have laminitis - his soles are just super sensitive. Consequently he now has pads that cover the soles completely and is shod every 4-5 weeks.

Initially he seemed interested in quite a few oils, however when they were offered again later on that day he had no further interest in any of the oils other than the arnica macerated oil, which has kept him sound. He goes off it for a while and then wants its healing properties again, just when his owner notices that he is getting 'footy'. He was beginning to feel his feet just before his owner went on holiday for a month. He wasn't ridden during this time so no arnica was offered, as he was just turned out with a small amount of lunging. On her return he was very sore and couldn't wait to have some arnica macerate which he kept nudging her for as soon as he thought she might take it away. Within a few days he was totally sound and competing again.

Eye injury
Dida Wales 2006

One day in late March I came home to find my horse, 'Flash' minus a shoe, covered in scratches, with a nasty cut to his left eye. I am not sure what he'd been getting up to, but I expect it started out as a game, and left him feeling very sorry for himself. He was waiting for me when I got back and it was clear that the eye was sore and he was quite upset.

Traditionally damage to the eye is something you don't take any chances with, previously we called the vet for a prior encounter with a tree. His treatment and advice was to check the eye itself wasn't damaged in any way, then to administer an anti-inflammatory, antibiotic and analgesic jab followed by advice to clean the area, and apply aloe-vera gel to the damaged skin tissue.

I cleaned up the area as best as I could and checked there was nothing in the eye. I then offered numerous oils for Flash to select. He chose rose, yarrow, juniper berry, frankincense, carrot seed, peppermint, arnica macerate, comfrey macerate and devil's claw tuber.

I offered him aloe gel and he nuzzled it, so I added some yarrow and applied it round the eye. He was stained very blue! He wanted a lot of macerates and devil's claw, licked heavily at the yarrow and carrot seed and inhaled other oils. He took these remedies three times a day for four days, as well as having the yarrow aloe gel applied copiously around the eye. During this time Flash would often come and find me for a cuddle and sympathy as well.

After day four he looked much better and the swelling had gone down considerably. He no longer asked for the oils, but was happy to have the gel applied twice a day. The area was healing up nicely, although he still wanted attention. I continued with the gel for another week and re-offered the oils again. He again wanted arnica macerate, which he took twice a day for a further two days.

Authors Note: Usually sandalwood or cornflower water are selected for eye problems, however the former applies to infection and the latter to congenital problems. In this case yarrow was appropriate as it related to a wound and inflammation.

Canine

In the wild a dog's staple food would probably be made up of animals such as rabbit with the contents of the gut providing them their quoter of plant materials. Perhaps this is why the macerates are so popular, because they offer similar important plant components with natural oils, both of which are lacking in the diets of most domesticated dogs. Offering remedies that are similar to those they may find in the wild such as the macerates, beeswax and spirulina have provided astonishing results.

Dogs are normally drawn to floral essential oils which are usually taken by inhalation, however, they do choose to sometimes lick essential oils but will generally only take very small amounts. The heavier oils are usually favoured for licking such as the absolutes, seabuckthorn, the macerates and spirulina. Essential oils rich in monoterpenes volitise rapidly into to the air, which unless offered slowly, may cause the dog to turn away at the intensity of the aroma; a needed oil may then be misread as not needed.

You will find that dogs often appear quite bashful and shy after inhalation, or lay down with their head in between their front paws. They may then lick the lower part of their front leg as if applying some form of accupressure to themselves.

Remedies frequently selected by dogs

Essential oils and extracts

Angelica root

Bergamot

Chamomile German

Chamomile Roman

Frankincense

Jasmine

Linden blossom

Lotus pink

Neroli

Peppermint

Rosehip - very popular

Rose otto

Sandalwood

Seaweed -very popular

Thyme

Valerian

Vetiver

Violet leaf

Yarrow

Yellow birch

Ylang ylang

Aromatic waters: Cornflower - very popular

Macerated oils: All very popular

Other remedies

Beeswax in a fixed oil (popular for infection)

Chalk powder - mixed with a fixed oil

Clay

Spirulina (very popular)

Fixed oils

Grapeseed

Sunflower

Olive

Number of each generally selected

3-4 essential oils and extracts

3-4 macerated oils

Dried remedies such as chalk and spirulina

Cornflower water

What to do if a dog appears to like all the macerated oils equally

A dog's diet is often lacking in natural oils, so it could be that macerated oils are selected for their fatty content and not for the plant material macerated in it. If a dog seems interested in all the oils offered, perform a test by offering a fixed oil such as grapeseed, sunflower or olive oil and assess how keen the dog is by:

- how quickly the tongue licks the oil off the hand
- whether every last trace is licked off the hand
- the urgency of the licking

Then offer the preferred selected macerated oils, re - run the above test and assess the difference as to which type of oil is actually needed. If the dog shows the same interest in them, work with the fixed oils first. After a while the dog will take much smaller amounts. When its interest wanes go back to offering the macerates However if you feel that your dog will greatly benefit from any of the macerates, then also work with them.

When deciding which oils are preferred, watch for every detail. Some dogs will be easier to assess than others. If you are finding this difficult, email the address at the back of this book for advice.

Macerated and fixed oils, in my experience, will not cause diarrhoea. In fact, carrot macerate has been known to be effective in treating diarrhoea. Sometimes a dog takes so much oil on the first offering that it is sick; this may equate to using the oil to purge toxins from the body as with eating grass. This appears to happen infrequently and is not often repeated

Note: Sourcing the oils for their fat content alone does not appear to be the case with horses and cats.

An example of a dog taking large quantities of macerated oils and fixed oils by Lottie Mattess

I have selected this study as it demonstrates a dog taking large quantities of base oils, much greater than those suggested in this book. It is interesting to note that on the second day, Xena took considerably more oils than on the first day.

Xena a two and a half year old short - haired German Shepherd, had for the last ten days been constantly licking her hind paw, between the pads. There did not seem to be any foreign objects in the paw, however the inside was red and irritated and she had almost removed the top layer of skin by licking. Xena also suffered from sore ears, especially after playing in water. These became red and itchy with a build up of brown wax, which according to the vet was a form of yeast infection in the ear. Xena also had a tendency to whine.

Xena began by taking small quantities of the oils recorded on the next page, which were then increased considerably over the following weeks.

Remedies offered daily

7th April 2004 - 7th June 2004

Day 1: Morning 07.04.04

Cornflower water	drank 90 mls
Angelica root	moderate interest, easily distracted
Rose otto	interested
Yarrow	stretch, lay down eyes heavy
Neroli	whined after inhaling (not an uncommon response to neroli)
German chamomile	slight thought
Roman chamomile	nodding off

Afternoon

Calendula CO_2	licked 2 mls
Carrot macerate	no interest
Grapeseed fixed oil	licked 2 mls
Apricot kernel	licked 2 mls
Spirulina	loves this

Day 2: Morning

Cornflower water	drank 90 mls
Calendula CO_2	licked 20 mls
Chickweed	licked 50 mls
Carrot macerate	licked 5 mls
Grapeseed fixed oil	licked 20 mls
Apricot kernel	licked 20 mls
Spirulina	finished bowl. Coat noticeably shinier than yesterday.

Xena had a total 115ml of vegetable and herbal oils today. As she wanted so much they were put into a bowl as opposed to being licked off the hand. She continued with a similar pattern over the days to follow.

10 days later

Xena was still selecting large quantities

Cornflower water	drank 40 mls
Chickweed	licked 105 mls
Grapeseed	none
Spirulina	Finished bowl

14 days later

Sandalwood	Slight lick
Chickweed	licked 80 mls
Grape seed	licked 90 mls
Spirulina	Finished bowl

Over the days Xena keenly selected rose otto, seaweed extract, neroli, yarrow and angelica. This continued for about a month. She then gradually selected less and less and by the end of the second month, Xena was no longer taking any remedies, except for spirulina, which she only took on some days. 'This was a very positive experience for both myself and Xena as she no longer has a problem with her ears or itchy paw. Over all it was a great result for Xena who now also has a lovely soft shiny coat. I found it fascinating to watch Xena and her reactions to the oils, which is a 'language' all of its own.

Remedies for common problems

Wounds

Yarrow

Use on broken skin and in conditions where pus exudes from the wound. It is a powerful anti-inflammatory and helps to reduce swelling, sooth inflamed tissues and neutralise excess heat and pain. Yarrow provides an environment where it is difficult for bacteria to grow. It also helps to release the trauma associated with the wound so could be used as a rescue remedy.

Use yarrow undiluted on open wounds. Apply drops to the wound until the area stains blue. The wound will absorb the amount needed before it stains. For larger areas add yarrow to an aloe vera gel.

Carrot seed

Carrot seed controls excessive bleeding (especially internal). It is indicated for internal damage for its cell-stimulating and repair properties.

Sea buckthorn or lavender

Enhances the formation of cell tissue and is useful where there is scar tissue. Use undiluted or in an aloe gel.

Seaweed

Protects and seals the wound, draws out impurities and prevents the invasion of foreign bodies. Seaweed contains iodine, an antiseptic; sulphur, noted for its blood purifying and antibacterial action; magnesium for nerve function, and zinc, renowned for its wound-healing and immune stimulating properties. Use undiluted or in aloe gel.

Dead Sea mud and clay

These can be used on their own for wounds. The clay can be made into a paste by adding water or sprinkled dry onto a oozing wound. Many animals in the wild are seen to use mud to help heal wounds.

Offer arnica and rose for shock

First aid wound gel
Yarrow 6 drops
Seaweed 1ml (20/30 drops)
Mix together in 50ml aloe vera gel.

Ear infections

Remedies are not usually applied topically to the ear, however yarrow and or German chamomile in a gel applied around the ear, not in the ear should be fine and can really help the problem, bringing relief to the area.

Remedies taken by mouth usually work well. The most popular is beeswax in a selected macerated or fixed oil, such as rosehip or grapeseed oil. To this you can add a couple of drops of thyme essential oil, or rosehip extract, depending on which is selected. Also offer orally spirulina, sandalwood, sea buckthorn, and remedies to support both the immune system and the emotional body.

Arthritis, joint / ligament problems and inflammation

The remedies below may produce astounding results. Spirulina and fixed or macerated oils are particular favourites with many dogs with joint problems. To begin with large quantities from the 'remedy list' are often selected.

Remedies to offer (usually taken orally)

Arnica	bruising / shock
Chalk powder	joint / bone disorders (calcium)
Chamomile German	inflammation
Comfrey	inflammation / pulled muscles / tendons and ligaments
Cornflower water	selected after operation / joint problems
Hemp	arthritis / joint problems / immune deficiency
Seaweed gel	repair / lack of movement
Spirulina	repair (very popular)
Yarrow	inflammation

Oils to offer for a gel: where there is heat or swelling

Chamomile German	tissue anti-inflammatory
Peppermint	anti-inflammatory (deep heat / cooling effect)
Juniper	fluid retention / arthritis
Birch	analgesic / deep heat / warming / healing
Yarrow	tissue anti-inflammatory
Immortelle	bruising / cell regenerating
Marjoram	anti-spasmodic / soothing
Valerian	deep muscle relaxant

Offer the selected oils orally and add appropriate ones to a gel.

Add a total of 25-50 drops of essential oil to 150 ml of aloe gel, depending on the severity of the condition.

Application

Apply to the affected area 1-2 x daily or as needed. Reduce the frequency of the application as the dog indicates. Allow to lick the gel from the hand.

Pain relief / anti-inflammatory gel

Peppermint   15 - 30 drops
Yarrow   4 - 6 drops
Birch   7 - 15 drops (depending on severity and the size of the dog)
Blend into 150 ml gel.

Application

Offer each oil to decide which to put into the gel. The dogs keenness and condition will help you decide on how many drops to add, the above suggestions are a guide line. Before each application offer the remedy. Apply to the affected area 1-2 x daily or as needed. Reduce the frequency of the application as the dog indicates. Allow them to lick the gel from the hand.

Skin Problems

Many dogs suffer from unbearable itchy skin and these remedies suggested are capable of offering much needed relief. Offer the ones that would be appropriate, then add them to a gel. Gels usually offer instant relief. For hot areas such as on the hind back, just above the tail, apply peppermint in a gel. Ringo, a German Shepherd with 'hot skin', would go up to his bottle of peppermint gel and push his nose against it whenever he wanted some applied - after its application he would then run friskily around the garden. Peppermint and German chamomile (great mugwort if the condition is very bad) will often relieve itching almost immediately. It is important to also check your dogs diet as along with vaccine reactions, this can be a contributing factor to skin problems.

The macerates and spirulina are invaluable for dogs with dermal problems, often providing miraculous results. These are normally taken in large amounts over a period of time, usually two weeks to two months.

Itchy irritated / inflamed / bald patches: topical gel (may be licked)

German chamomile	7 drops	inflamed skin / antihistamine
Roman chamomile	7 drops	bald patches / anxiety
Peppermint	30 drops	hot or itchy skin
Sandalwood	5 - 7 drops	dry skin

Add selected oil or oils to 150ml watery aloe vera gel.

Also offer: Oral / inhalation

The remedies listed below are also important for skin problems.

Flax oil
Hemp oil
Marigold macerated oil / extract
Rosehip macerate oil
Sea buckthorn extract
Seaweed
Spirulina

Application

Offer the remedy to the dog before each application. Apply to the affected areas daily or as needed. Allow them to lick the gel if they choose to.

Hot skin: Pour on hand; run through the coat.
Inflamed skin: Apply directly to effected areas.
Stubborn/raw areas may need German chamomile applied undiluted.

Note: Skin disorders are very often associated with diet or vaccines which have been known to cause auto immune sensitive responses.

Tumours / warts / lumps

The treatment of tumours and warts is not always straightforward. As with most conditions the behavioural element needs to be addressed together with the symptoms. Oils to support the liver and kidneys, the primary organs for cleansing the body and oils for the immune system should also be considered.

Offer for inhalation / orally
Angelica root (not seed)
Bergamot - frequently selected
Grapefruit (especially popular with dogs that have fatty lumps)

Caution: the above oils are photo-reactive.

Also frequently selected are seaweed extract and spirulina which help support the liver and bodily function.

Application
Topically the oils can be applied in an aloe gel. Apply daily or as needed.

Travelling

Many animals suffer from car sickness especially when young. Plenty of fresh air and good visibility are important but in addition you may want to offer the following:

Bergamot	balancing
Black currant bud	balancing / refreshing
Carrot seed	supports the liver
Camomile Roman	anxiety / stomach
Lime	stomach / liver
Peppermint	settles the stomach
Spirulina / chalk / clay	settles the stomach

In Chinese medicine the kidneys relate to the ears and balance. It may also be worth while offering oils to support the kidneys since car sickness is often related to balance.

Offer the aromas before travel and then again at the start of the journey, also try stopping a few minutes after setting off to offer selected oils.

Gum disease / toothpaste

A raw food diet should prevent tooth and gum disorders. However, if problems arise make up and offer the following:

30 g green clay (detoxifies)
10 g chalk (supports teeth)
2 drops peppermint (cleansing)
1-2 drops of thyme (infection)
Mix together and shake well.

Application
Offer the remedy. Apply with the fingers to the gums, providing the animal lets you. Never hold the head to apply. **Caution:** Dogs that bite!

Case studies: canine

Hip dysplasia
Donna Scotter 2005

Storm is a 9 year old black and tan German Shepherd. At six months old he was diagnosed with hip dysplasia, which results from an abnormal development in the ball and socket joint of the hip. The condition is degenerative and can cause pain, lameness and osteoarthritis. We went through all the usual procedures of radiographs and various consultations and were told that there was nothing that could be done until Storm was fully matured. At this stage they would suggest an operation to cut certain muscles around the hip joints to help reduce the pain he was in. However, when he was fully grown his condition was thought to be so severe that any operation would be pointless. We were advised to manage his condition through controlled exercise and pain management with anti-inflammatory medication. I was not happy for Storm to be on medication for the rest of his life and Storm was not happy to give up walks. But what choice did we have?

Storm is normally a warm, gentle, affectionate dog, however, in recent years he has become grumpy especially after exercise or in colder weather, which to me points to his to being in pain. At around three years of age I replaced his medication with homeopathic arnica, which at first helped to relieve his pain, but as time went on his mobility became increasingly restricted. He could no longer jump into the back of the car and would have to be wheel barrowed up the steps to our house. His back end was very weak and his bones made a crunching sensation when massaged (which he loved). When I became a student at the Institute of Animal Aromatics, Storm was one of my first case studies.

The oils he selected were

Cornflower water: Opens up to healing/ soporific
Rose otto: Trauma and resentment
Jasmine: Hormone balancer, comforting
Comfrey: Anti-inflammatory, damaged tendons, ligaments and bones
Spirulina: Aids in cell repair / immune responses
Peppermint: Stimulates blood / nerve function
St John's wort: Nerve damage, antidepressant

I also made up 25 ml diluted aloe vera gel and added 10 drops of peppermint and 8 drops of helichrysum (which Storm inhaled). This was massaged into his hips daily. Following his initial treatment with the gel whenever Storm saw me getting my oil box out he bounded over to me. Three weeks into his remedies, we decided to go away in our caravan. What we experienced next with him was unbelievable. Storm jumped into the car unaided and played with the younger dogs all the time we were away, then when we returned he climbed the stairs to our house all on his own. His bones no longer crunched when we massage his hips and he is back to his old personality. With other dogs he acts like a puppy and no longer growls under his breath at the kids.

Storm was my first success story and whilst I realise I cannot cure him, if I help to slow down the degeneration to his hip joints (even regenerate them to a certain extent) and provide him with pain relief, he will be a much happier dog.

A Jack Russell Terrier with degenerative back problems
Penny Ward 2006

Poppy has health problems and her owner felt she had given up the will to survive. When Poppy was two 2 years old she chased a cat and went under a gate. Her front end went through but her hindquarters got stuck. Her back was broken and she became paralysed from the middle of her back down. She had an operation where the vertebrae in her spine were fused together, but it took several months before she made a full recovery.

Her temperament is like that of a normal Jack Russell - fun loving, playful and lively. However, in the last six months (now at the age of 10), she has become very slow and stiff in her rear end and cannot use her hind legs to their full extent, so drags them around after her. She has to be picked up to go outside to relieve herself and is beginning to lose sensation in her hind end, causing her to mess in the house. The vet prescribed a very strong medication to mix into her food, but Poppy had become very 'down in the dumps' and appeared to be losing the will to live. Her owner fears that it would be kinder to put her to sleep.

Selected remedies:
Rose otto: 3 sniffs
Rose absolute: inhalation, went away, lay down and was thoughtful, eyelids lowering. Came back, had four more inhalations
Yarrow : 2 deep inhalations
Bergamot: no reaction
Peppermint: 3 very deep long inhalations and then a grunt and a squeal!
Wintergreen: lots of little sniffs, then walked away for a while, lay down in thought
Carrot seed: no reaction
Roman chamomile: inhalation - that was enough
Comfrey: No reaction
St John's wort: no reaction
Arnica macerate: huge reaction

Arnica macerated oil: I poured about a teaspoonful into my hand, which Poppy licked off and then begged for more. I only gave her very small amounts due to caution being advised. However, when I offered her more from the hand she licked it all up and was frantic to get more. We observed her for a while and she showed no adverse signs and was keen for more. She was running around us in little circles, making squealing noises and jumping up at the bottle of arnica.

Her owner was amazed at Poppy's reaction to the macerated oil. As the arnica is macerated in olive oil the owner suggested that it might actually be the fatty oils that are needed and not the arnica. So Poppy was offered olive oil on its own, which she showed no interest in at all. The owner then offered Poppy more arnica oil, which she eagerly licked up, still wanting more. In all she had about 4-6 teaspoonfuls.

The owner was left with rose absolute, yarrow, peppermint and arnica to offer Poppy and was made aware of the safety implications regarding the arnica. After several days the essential oils were no longer taken, but she still continued to take the arnica macerated oil. Initially, over the first four days she was taking a tablespoon a day, then she only wanted it every other day. After about a week she had half a tablespoon every 3 - 4 days, this continued for about 2 months. When Poppy first started taking arnica she would go and sit under the cupboard where the bottle was kept and make little squealing noises. The first time she did this the owner was not sure what was wrong with Poppy so asked her what the matter was, opened the kitchen door to see if she needed to go out and got her treats to see if she wanted them (she did!) but still she sat under the cupboard squealing. Her owner opened the cupboard door and Poppy became very excited, wagging her tail indicating that she wanted the arnica macerate. As time went on over the two months she did this less and less but always indicated to her owner when she wanted the arnica oil.

Since taking her remedies, Poppy has a new lease of life and this has thrilled her owners. She has a lot more energy and her mood has completely changed from being somewhat depressed to being bright and alert. She is a lot less stiff, especially in her back and hind legs and as a result is more active. Her coat is glossy, her eyes are no longer dull and she seems to have her old spirit back. Members of the family and friends have remarked on the change in her.

A whippet with a puncture wound
Donna Scotter 2003

A recent visit from the postman caused mayhem in the house with all three of my dogs underfoot. Patch overstepped the mark, Milo nipped him to put him in his place and a full scale dog fight ensued. Milo received a small puncture wound in his chest at the top of his leg and he was limping. After a few hours the limp got worse and the area around the wound became swollen and hot to touch. I offered Milo remedies, even if only to help with the shock from the fight.

I offered yarrow for the inflammation and emotional release (rescue remedy), which he inhaled several times then turned away to process it. I also offered lavender, German chamomile, peppermint and wintergreen and no interest was shown in any of them. I have subsequently found that usually yarrow, rose and arnica are selected when an animal is first wounded. Finally, I offered him carrot seed for cell repair. He loved it, first he inhaled it and then I added some to sunflower oil and he licked it off my hand.

I made up 25ml of diluted aloe vera gel and added 10 drops each of carrot seed and yarrow. I applied this to Milo's chest and shoulder every two hours and before he went to bed that night. The next morning there was no limp, no swelling and no heat, and Milo showed no further interest in any of the oils.

A prostate-prompted problem
Jan Wilmot: 2006 Santa Fe New Mexico

Snoop is a 10 year old retired working Cocker Spaniel, he lost an eye to glaucoma about a year ago and is largely deaf, so is now living as a house dog.

While I was visiting a friend in America, Snoop was taken ill. He had an upset stomach but was straining so hard that he appeared to be developing piles and was constantly licking his anal area, which looked very sore and swollen causing him to get quite distressed. Initially I found some aloe in a cupboard and his owner applied a little to his anal area, which was so painful that he was growling quietly at her and really did not want it touched. As I was travelling I did not have many oils with me, but with the vets closed for a holiday weekend and no emergency cover available I felt that I had to do something more for him. Having seen his reaction I knew he was so sore that it would be difficult if not impossible to put anything further directly on the area.

I thought that the most likely available oil to be of interest would be peppermint, so offered this in the bottle, which provoked a licking reaction. I then found some flax oil in the cupboard and offered that, which was accepted. I mixed about 1 tablespoon of flax oil with 4 drops of peppermint and this was eagerly licked up. I made up this mix again four times by which time he was a little less desperate for it but appeared to be trying to get it on himself, so I dabbed a very small amount on his chest and he went to doze with his nose firmly on the scent. Whilst he was still 'looking' at his rear end every now and then, the distressed licking stopped immediately. The following day he appeared to be much better, with the swelling round his anal area much reduced and a healthier pink. I reoffered the peppermint in flax oil, which he licked half heartedly, taking only 1 tablespoonful. By lunch time when more was offered he had no interest in it at all and his anal area was back to normal size and a healthy looking pink.

Nervous urinating
Caroline Ingraham 2006

Harry is a miniature, long haired dachshund aged six and half years. He came to us when he was 12 weeks of age. Shortly after he arrived we became concerned at the appearance of his eyes. We asked the vet to check them and he finally announced that Harry had retinal degeneration and would be blind by the time he was two years old. We have now since discovered that he is a carrier of the condition but will not go blind, however his eyesight problems have made him inclined to be nervous. For example, he would jump if there was anything on the floor that he did not expect, such as a cushion, growling nervously.

When we moved house we had to change vets. On the first visit Harry was very nervous and had a bowel action and urinated on the table. On the next visit to the surgery, to be neutered, I stayed with him while his sedative began to take effect. Unfortunately, a loud noise startled him and made him leap up frantically, causing the vet to quickly grab hold of him and cage him. The following year we decided to change vets and told the new vet, of our past experience. She suggested that we bring Harry into the surgery without anything done to him other than being offered a treat (which he always refused) so he would perceive it as a positive experience. Despite many visits to the vets, sometimes simply walking in and out with him there was only minimum improvement. Each time it would result in him messing on the table. The following year I decided to learn Reiki and used it to help Harry. On the next vet visit he did actually stand without a great struggle, albeit with a terrified look on his face, and he still messed on the table.

Examples of things that made him nervous
- If someone (even us) bends down to pat him he will jump and shriek as if he has been hurt, even if no contact is made. At other times he will come up to us wanting to be stroked.
- Sometimes when I suggest a walk he simply decides he is too afraid to go, and no amount of firmness, bribing, cajoling or eagerness from me will persuade him. At this time he frequently inspects himself to check that he is not urinating. If we leave him he is distressed and when we return he is likely to pass small amounts of urine.
- If ever he is nervous about anything he checks that he is not passing urine. Interestingly though, he will go for long periods in the car without the need to urinate.
- He will bark at anything he is worried about and check himself. He does this even when people he knows come into the house.

The following oils were selected
Cornflower water
Frankincense diluted in water
Neroli diluted in water
Yarrow diluted in olive oil
Jasmine diluted in olive oil
Arnica macerated oil
Hemp macerated oil
Rosehip fruit extract
Spirulina

Update: Morning oils
Hemp: very interested to start with, then just a quick smell.

Arnica: very interested each time. Tail wagging, leans over to sniff more than once, swallows and sticks tongue out and in. Sits with heavy eyelids nose twitching.

Rosehip: started with moderate interest, then low interest.

Spirulina: offered it to him in water and he took 10 licks in spurts. The following day he was not interested in it offered in water, so I made it up into a paste using half teaspoonful. He stood by my side waiting for it and then took most of it!

Update: Evening oils
Cornflower oil: has moved from a keen interest, licking about 20 mls, down to 4 mls then 3 mls to just one lick with nose twitching.

Neroli: started with a very tentative sniff, nose twitching and a whine. Now a more confident sniff, nose twitching.

Yarrow: started off by trying to lick it but recoiled away. The following day he sniffed, snorted and then became disinterested in it. In the days to follow there was moderate interest with nose twitching. However last night he began to open up to it, so long as it was not placed too near - licking, swallowing wagging tail, whining, nose twitching.

Jasmine: started with short interest, lick and a grumble, then for the next two nights he was less interested, until last night when he became more responsive, twitching his nose, licking and swallowing.

Frankincense: started off eagerly, concentrating on its aroma. Followed by two days of minimal interest, then last night, as with the yarrow and jasmine he showed a greater interest, taking it in with nose twitching, and tail wagging.

His behaviour is, I feel, improving. We have had two visitors, which would have entailed him to bark beyond necessity. This time he stopped as soon as I indicated for him to do so, and did not continue grumbling as usual. We have not had any sudden nervous yelps from him over the past few days, but I feel a bit more time is needed to prove that he is cured, although he is much more relaxed. I noticed that when he wanted to get the position of one of the other dogs he just did it and stood his ground, which I don't think he would have done previously. The real test for me will be to take him to the vets!

2nd Update

Well what a week! A couple of days before we went away in our motor van Harry became very tense and nervous again. I couldn't understand why he had changed back. He refused to get in the van, then he would not come out and then he whined for most of the journey. When we stopped, thinking he might want to pass urine, again he would not get out. He eventually shot out and I had to quickly catch him, which made him shriek. I was really at my wits end with him. However, later that day I noticed a wet patch on his hind quarters and when I checked I found he has an abscess on his bottom - a good reason to be miserable! The next morning I took him to the local vet (having to take him to a strange vet was my worst nightmare come true). I dabbed arnica on his paw and gave him several sniffs of frankincense before and during our wait in the surgery. When we got in he was as calm as can be, I could hardly believe it! He stood on the table and I was fully expecting him to make it very difficult for the vet to see the abscess, by trying to tuck his tail under. However, he let me gently hold up his tail and allowed the examination with only a small shout when the abscess was touched. So what a test!!! Also while we were in the surgery he allowed two people to stroke him without a murmur - a complete difference from his previous behaviour.

He still continues the oils with interest, but not prolonged inhalations. The arnica still is high on his list and the frankincense is less, but he is now more interested in rose. Thanks for all your help, we can certainly see a vast improvement in Harry.

Runny eyes
Tamara Roberts 2005

Coral is nearly two and since she was a puppy has had runny eyes. The vet could find nothing wrong - it wasn't conjunctivitis and her tear ducts weren't blocked. Muscle testing suggested weakness in the liver and eyes (in Chinese medicine the liver and eyes are connected). The remedies that were indicated were peppermint, bergamot, sandalwood, cornflower water and spirulina.

Peppermint and bergamot were diluted in a base oil and offered for Coral to inhale or lick. Sandalwood was diluted in water and offered both for inhalation and to lick, this was also gently wiped across her eyes. Cornflower water was offered to inhale or lick. Coral seemed to prefer the spirulina without any water. After two days Coral lost interest in peppermint and bergamot. On the fifth, sixth and seventh days of offering the remedies changes to the discharge were noticeable and there was more weeping. Coral then lost interest in all of the remedies other than the spirulina. She became noticeably quieter and I thought she may be having a 'healing crisis'.

Following what appeared to be a 'healing crisis' she regained interest in cornflower water, sandalwood and spirulina for a period of eight days before showing a gradual disinterest in everything except the spirulina. Then suddenly, overnight, Coral's eyes stopped weeping and she became bright and playful, as though feeling good in herself.

Hip and elbow dysplasia
Torie Broomhead 2006

Beau is a 15 month old black Labrador who was diagnosed with hip and elbow dysplasia when he was just 6 months old.

From a young age Beau showed signs of lameness, discomfort and depression. He was unable to interact with other puppies, climb stairs and he often cried in pain during the night. Beau underwent a number of x-rays and hip manipulations to find out the severity of his condition. The x-rays showed that Beau's condition was very serious and his options were limited. The vet suggested that he should be referred to a specialist to consider a total hip replacement; however, it would not be advisable for Beau to have the operation until he was at least 1 year old and fully grown.

In the meantime the vet prescribed him a painkiller known as Norocarp to help him feel more comfortable, and a course of injections which he would have weekly to try and prevent the early stages of arthritis. After a couple of weeks on painkillers and injections, Beau's behaviour took a turn for the worst, he seemed even more depressed and his energy levels dropped dramatically. I decided that the painkillers were not making Beau happy and that he was better off without them. After a lot of thought I also decided that the hip replacement was not the answer either, as it involved a lot of risks and it was such a major operation for a young dog. I then researched complementary therapy and came across Caroline's course, so I decided to enroll as a student to see if I could learn more to help Beau.

During the first weekend of the course Caroline offered Beau Spirulina and comfrey macerated oil. Beau showed a lot of interest in them, so Caroline mixed 1 tablespoon of spirulina with water to form a watery paste. Beau took one sniff and ate every last bit, so Caroline offered some more to see if he was still interested and he ate that even faster. Over the four days he consumed at least 100g of spirulina and around 300 mls of macerated oils along with other remedies such as rosehip extract and sea buckthorn, as well as inhaling and licking various essential oils. During the course Beau was like a different dog. He was racing around the garden chasing after my other puppy and for the first time ever I couldn't catch him!

Beau was feeling great and he continued to show improvement with a lot more energy, he also looked a lot happier. A few months on and Beau is still doing well, he is still a lot happier and can manage much longer walks without being stiff the following day. Beau continues to select spirulina and comfrey oil since the course (five months ago), and he is now also selecting seaweed carrageen gel, beeswax and chalk mixed into a fixed oil. Beau is also fed a holistic diet of raw meat, fruit, vegetables and bones to keep him slim and healthy.

Itchy skin
Janet Mortimer

I was attending the first part of my Animal Aromatics course with Caroline and was staying in Hay-on-Wye with my two dogs Caspar and Cleo. Caspar is an eight year old greyhound. I've had him since he was six months old and from time to time he has a problem with itchy skin. I've never been able to work out what triggers the reaction and the symptoms vary slightly each time. It doesn't appear to be diet related but could possibly be linked to insects or grasses in the summer. My studying was going fine but then Caspar suddenly seemed to have a terrible problem with his skin. All of the lower part of his stomach and between his back legs became extremely inflamed, hot and red looking. Poor Caspar didn't know what to do with himself, he couldn't relax or sit still, and he was biting himself making his skin very sore. In desperation I asked Caroline if I could bring Caspar to the class to see if she could help him. He proved himself an excellent subject for the students and myself to observe! Almost as soon as he started inhaling oils he appeared to be much calmer. He selected marigold macerated oil, great mugwort, peppermint and yarrow. He wasn't interested in spirulina. He took lots of marigold macerate - possibly as much as 40 ml, avidly licking it from my hand and between my fingers making sure he got every last drop. It seemed to send him into an almost trance like state, with a glazed expression, as he processed it. Great mugwort, peppermint and yarrow were added to aloe vera gel to help his skin become less hot and itchy. He was so pleased to have it applied, he laid on his back with his legs spread wide to help me. His keen interest in marigold macerate lasted for several days, this he took in quite large quantities each time it was offered. His interest in the gel continued for about three days, by which time the scratching had stopped and his skin was nearly back to normal.

Since then Caspar hasn't had a problem with his skin again. He's always really interested in my box of oils and happy to sample them. The macerated and fixed oils are usually his favourites, but by no means all of them. He still enjoys marigold and also likes chickweed and hemp.

Fear of Fireworks
Tamara Roberts

Woody is a golden Labrador owned by Animal Aromatics graduate Tamara Roberts. Generally he is a confident dog, however, on fireworks night he becomes anxious and paces. Tam offered him the following remedies all of which he selected: cornflower water, frankincense, valerian, vetiver, sandalwood, lavender and violet leaf. His favourites were vetiver and lavender which he inhaled deeply and licked. Despite the fireworks, within five minutes he was asleep.

Feline

Since cats do not have metabolic pathways to break down essential oils, it is thought that they should not be offered. After reading the studies in this book, you may agree that denying these remedies would be a great loss to the cat, however, working with essential oils and cats is a little more difficult than with other animals. Generally cats are very sensitive to essential oils, and the range of remedies they select is much fewer than those selected by herbivores, which eat plants as part of their diet. A cat will select a plant for its medicinal value only; they do not have the enzymes to readily metabolise and get rid of unwanted plant compounds, but cats are able to cope with the plant oils that they require. The importance lies in reading the cats' response to the aromas and not forcing any on them. An unwanted essential oil can be relatively toxic to a cat, and an aroma that is not needed, can make a cat very wary of other essential oil bottles.

Essential oils are not generally applied to cats topically, and they are not usually taken by mouth, except topical preparations such as flea powder with peppermint, clay and chalk. Heavier remedies such as seaweed and rosehip extract should not present a problem, they are also selected by cats orally. Macerates, especially chickweed are very popular and often licked, especially by cats with skin conditions. The macerates would perhaps be similar to what a cat would find in the gut of its kill. Clay works well as a poultice on their wounds, which again may be a behaviour simular to that practiced in the wild.

Remedies frequently selected by cats

Angelica root
Arnica flowers macerated oil
Cedarwood
Chickweed macerated oil
Cornflower water
Elemi
Frankincense
Hemp macerated oil
Lavender
Lemon
Linden blossom absolute
Lotus - pink
Marigold macerated oil
Neroli
Patchouli
Rosehip extract
Rose otto and absolute
Sandalwood
Sea buckthorn CO_2
Seaweed extract
Spikenard
Valerian
Violet leaf absolute
Wheatgrass powder
Yarrow

Note: Essential oils are generally selected for inhalation only.

Other remedies:

Clay (wounds and flea powder)
Dead Sea mineral mud
Dried catnip, rose and peppermint
Spirulina

Fixed oils

Sunflower
Olive

Number of each generally selected

3-5 essential oils
3-5 macerated oils and extracts
Dried remedies such as clay and catnip flowers

How to offer remedies to cats

The best time to read a cats responses to the aromas, is when the remedies are offered at a time when they are quiet and settled, or when they are in a 'pet carrier'.

Slowly approach the cat with the aroma. When you see its head begin to turn away, stop - this will be the distance required for the aroma molecules. The cat will now most likely be in trance like state and hold its position. If you feel after a while that more is needed go closer. Your cat will choose its distance from the aroma thus guiding its dosage.

Cats are smart, they will not take anything they don't want! If they do not want the aroma they will turn away quickly or run from it.

If the aroma from the bottle is too strong, or they are suspicious of the bottles after inhaling an unwanted aroma, place a little on your fingertip (diluted if it is an essential oil) and gently introduce the new aroma that way. Other methods of working with cats include, lacing inspired remedies individually on cotton wool or cloth, they can then choose what time of day they want their remedies and how often.

Indoor cats

It is important to provide indoor cats as much stimulation as possible and make their environment as close to the outdoors as you can.

Indoor herbs and plants are always good but make sure they are not poisonous to cats. Peppermint, chickweed and catnip are generally popular herbs. You can also leave clean empty litter trays with dried herbs in, one for each herb. This way they can roll in them and behave as they would outside.

Popular dried herbs include:
Catnip
Chickweed
Peppermint
Rose petals
Valerian root

Remedies for common conditions

Grooming

A cat that had not groomed for 8 years, selected rose otto, immediately after inhaling it she frantically began grooming herself; this lasted a few minutes before her grooming calmed which she continued to do for the duration of the class that I was teaching. Rose otto can also be offered for over grooming.

Wounds

Cats appear to have no problem tolerating extracts such as seaweed and clay, in fact they respond incredibly well to their healing properties. To find out more about applying seaweed and clay to a wound refer to the 'Buzz' study.

Remedies to offer

Seaweed

Protects and seals the wound, draws out impurities and prevents the invasion of foreign bodies. It contains iodine, an antiseptic; sulphur, noted for its blood purifying and anti-bacterial action; magnesium for nerve function, and zinc, for its wound-healing and immune stimulating properties. Use in aloe gel or clay. (I have not yet tried it in Dead Sea mineral mud, which may also help a cat with wounds).

Dead Sea mud and clay

These can be used on their own for wounds. The clay can be made into a paste by adding water or simply sprinkled on to the wound to dry it out. I have only just began working with Dead Sea mineral mud, so at this stage I am not able to write much from experience as I have not yet used it with cats.

First aid wound gel

10 drops seaweed

Add to 50 ml aloe vera gel or green clay paste

Application

Offer the remedy to the cat. Apply as needed

Post wound gel

Sea buckthorn - undiluted / aloe gel / beeswax

Rosehip extract - undiluted / aloe gel / beeswax

Add selected remedies to a firm aloe vera gel. Otherwise a loose beeswax ointment

Application

Offer the remedy to the cat. Apply as needed.

Offer arnica macerated oil and rose for shock.

Thyroid problems

In a small animal veterinary practice where my clients were felines, I saw many hyperthyroid problems. The first cat was seventeen years old, she selected lavender, clear seaweed essential oil and seaweed absolute. On arrival her heart rate was high - 150, which is typical of a hyperthyroid cat, but within five minutes of inhaling the oils the heart rate normalised to 100.

Almost all cats with hyperthyroidism chose chickweed macerate, seaweed extract, and rose or lavender essential oil. In recent work with hyperthyroidism in cats, however, it has been noted that they will usually select spirulina.

Seaweed with its high iodine content would generally be considered for hypothyroidism (which is rare in cats). If it is selected it appears that it has a regulating effect on the thyroid, but if it is not selected it may cause problems.

Arthritis, joint / ligament problems and inflammation

Seaweed is probably the most popular remedy for mobility problems. In addition to the list below your cat may also choose to inhale other remedies. It would not be unusual for a cat to lick the macerated oils, spirulina, the seaweed and rosehip extract, wheatgrass powder or the cornflower water, even though they generally seem to treat themselves by inhalation.

Arnica	bruising / shock
Chickweed	rheumatic conditions
Comfrey	inflammation / pulled muscles / tendons and ligaments
Cornflower water	after an operation and where there are joint problems
Chamomile German	inflammation
Hemp	arthritis / joint problems / immune deficiency
Marigold	mimics the effects of certain steroids
Spirulina	cell repair (offer dry on finger tip)
Wheatgrass powder	cell repair (offer dry on finger tip)

Cystitis

The occurrence of cystitis in both male and female cats is very common.

Symptoms include

A frequent need to urinate and apparent discomfort

Only a few drops of urine passed at a time

Blood in the urine

Increased drinking of water

Constant scratching in the litter box, without passing urine

Whilst cystitis is normally caused by a bacterial infection in most species, with cats it is sometimes inconclusive as the urine samples are often sterile and the condition is commonly induced by stress. Kidney stones are another common cause, if this is thought to be the problem, offer lemon essential oil which is renowned for dissolving stones. If left untreated cystitis could lead to kidney infection, indicated by a high temperature and discomfort in the abdomen and lower back. Kidney infections can result in scarring and a decrease in kidney function. Is is important to ensure that your cat has a natural diet, water and exercise to help support the kidneys and ensure it does not become obese. This will give your cat the best chance of avoiding cystitis.

Refer to the case study on Tilly for selecting oils to help with cystitis. The inhalation alone of valerian works well for stress related cystitis, a case study on this by S. Davis can be found in 'A Step by Step Guide' under 'Examples of how the aroma alone can be effective'.

Case studies: feline

A bout of cystitis
Tamara Roberts 2005

Tilly has lived in her present home since she was eight weeks old. She is a little overweight but generally she is a healthy, contented cat, despite having previously suffered two bouts of cystitis and now showing symptoms again. She became agitated, struggling to urinate, spending a long time in her litter tray, yet only passing small amounts of strong smelling urine with some crystals and blood present. Antibiotics and anti-inflammatory drugs prescribed by a vet, had relieved these symptoms in the past but had not stopped them recurring. I decided to offer Tilly the following essential oils.

Essential oils for the kidneys

Juniper	fluid retention / detoxifies
Sandalwood	structural / antibacterial
Lemon	breaks down kidney stones
Lemon grass	cleansing
Yarrow	anti-inflammatory
Patchouli	eases bruising and swelling / antibacterial
Cedarwood	eases bruising and swelling / antibacterial
Carrot seed	cell repair

Tilly self-selected lemon, lemon grass and carrot seed. She appeared to enjoy these oils and whilst inhaling from the bottles she flicked her tail and purred. I offered her the oils, twice a day, for two days, and even though her symptoms ceased almost immediately, she continued to want carrot seed for another four days. Eight months later and Tilly is still free from further bouts of cystitis.

A nervous cat
Tamara Roberts 2004

Kin is a 6 year old Maine Coon rescue cat. She was originally found to have been cage reared and had not been socialised to people or environments, beyond the small carrier cage in which she was housed. She was discovered in an emaciated and ungroomed state. When Kin was first re-homed she was very wary of people and hid herself away, hissing at people if they got too close. She never achieved full size potential of her breed but is now in good condition. Kin is an indoor cat and still quite nervous. When not sleeping she repeatedly walks around her home environment. She does not really like physical contact with her owner, although she does like to sit close to her and follow her around the house. Kin does not actively play and does not like to be groomed or stroked.

When she was offered the oils she became quiet and rested, after which she was alert and interested, followed again by being very calm and relaxed, going into a trance like state.

Oils that were selected
Rose otto in water: five quick short sharp sniffs, ears laid back on head, appeared thoughtful.
Narcissus in grapeseed oil, one sniff then sprang backwards.
Bergamot in grapeseed oil: sniffed with ears laid back, pupils dilated, tail wagging, yawning.
St John's wort: one sniff, paused thoughtfully.
Wheat grass in grapeseed oil: sniffed, licked the air and walked away.
Carrot macerated oil: very keen and interested with several short shallow sniffs and a few pauses for thought. Tail wagging; she then paced around the room and came back to the oil again.

The essential oils were placed on cotton cloths as Kin was such a nervous cat.

Almost with immediate effect, Kin became noticeably calmer. Her owner reported that within a few days she jumped onto her lap and accepted gentle affectionate stroking, something that had been hoped for but previously never possible. She also let her owner groom her, which gave shine to her coat.

Kin has not shown any signs of timid or frightened behaviour since introducing her to the oils. She is behaving with far more confidence especially when visitors arrive in the house, prior to the oils she would have hid. Any changes to the owners daily routine would have caused Kin to become very distressed, she would then urinate on soft furnishings in the house, but to date there has been no evidence of this behaviour continuing.

This too is the first year that fireworks did not distress her, previously she hid as soon as she heard them, this year I am told that she appeared completely unaware of them. Kins owners are so happy with the changes in her behaviour, they now feel that they have a cat who is a pet rather than just a cat that lives in the home with them. All in all her owners seemed to have formed a much stronger bond with Kin and they are now considering constructing a secure garden where she can have access to the outside. In the meantime they have provide a tray lined with turf where Kin enjoys chewing on grass.

Wounded in a cat fight
Lottie Mattess 2004

Buzz came home and I could see he had been in a cat fight as he had scratches on his nose and ear. Upon checking him over I noticed a little scab on the top right hand side of his head. I decided to keep an eye on the scab, in case it turned into an abscess as they sometimes do.

Sure enough a few days later a lump was developing underneath the scab which I thought could be an abscess. The base of his right ear was also beginning to feel swollen and warm to the touch - another indication. I kept checking the area regularly to see if the lump/abscess had burst; it was about the size of a chickpea. Buzz could not lie on the right side of his head and was beginning to look a little put out, due to the discomfort. When the scab opened I saw a lot of pus sitting in the wound.

I let Buzz settle by the fire and while I gently squeezed and wiped away the thick green pus. A lot came out (about 1.5 mls), but Buzz was excellent and let me do this; it must have been a relief for him to have the pressure released, he began to purr. I rubbed his right ear in an upward direction to try and mobilise the pus. His fur was wet with pus and was getting in the way, so it was difficult to tell if I had cleaned it all out, so I decided to try a green clay poultice on the area and thought about adding some seaweed to amplify its drawing properties. I made up a small amount of green clay poultice by adding tepid spring water until it had a pasty consistency. I offered Buzz (who was still splayed out in front of the fire) clear and green seaweed, to see which one he preferred in his poultice, or indeed if he wanted anything at all!

He sniffed the clear (essential oil) seaweed, scrunched his eyes and face up, put his tongue out, then in and turned away. When I offered the green seaweed extract he stretched out to come to the oil, gave a very big, long deliberate sniff, followed by lots of tongue movement, catching the aromatic molecules in the air. He then lay his head down, looking at the bottle of green seaweed. So the green seaweed it was. I put 5 drops into 5 mls of the clay poultice and offered it to Buzz to see if he wanted to lick any. He had a little sniff but did not want any orally.

When I applied the poultice to the wound Buzz was chilled out and purring. I noticed after I had applied it that he lay on the right hand side of his head (the side of the wound), something he had not done since being injured.

Thirty minutes later when I checked the area I could see pus being drawn out into the green clay, so I wiped it off and applied more. I also decided to offer Buzz some bladderwrack (seaweed) powder, he did not want it dry, but had a few licks from the saucer when I added water. After a sleep he went out, and when he returned that evening I checked his wound, it was amazing! I could now see a little puncture hole where a tooth or a claw had caused the original injury to his head. There was no more pus to be seen. The skin around the hole was pink in colour and looked clean - not red and angry as it was before and the swelling around the wound had subsided dramatically. I tried gently squeezing the area to see if there was any more pus to come out, but no, it was definitely all gone, only clear fluid was visible.

I bathed the poultice off with warm water and cotton wool, and gently trimmed some of the surrounding fur away from the site of the wound to let the air get to it and help it heal. I was reluctant to leave the wound as it was but didn't want to interfere with it too much so decided to put a drop of neat, green seaweed extract on the hole to help it to heal and to form a protective barrier, preventing bacteria from entering. I again offered Buzz the green seaweed; he had a tiny sniff and turned away.

The next day I checked the area and it had scabbed over with a clear fluid and no sign of any blood. The swelling around the wound and at the base of his ear continued to reduce.

I next offered Buzz some bladderwrack powder mixed with spring water. He sniffed it and had four licks from the saucer, then walked off, indicating he had had enough.

Three days after treatment began, I checked Buzz again and his wound was healing nicely. The scab was intact, the swelling by the wound had completely gone and was much reduced by his ear, which by the fourth day was minimal and by day five there was no swelling anywhere. Buzz did not want any more bladderwrack powder or green seaweed. I could see pink new skin when parts of the scab come away and the puncture hole looked like it had long gone.

Conclusion

I'm over the moon that I was able to be of assistance in helping to heal Buzz's abscess myself with the aid of green clay, green seaweed extract CO_2 and the bladderwrack powder. The usual treatment at the vets when Buzz ends up in a fight and gets wounded in the same way is antibiotics and draining of pus. This involves at least two trips to the vet, causing Buzz further distress travelling and being in a strange place with strange smells etc.

With these natural remedies I have avoided the vet trips, but what I'm most pleased about is that Buzz did not need any antibiotics to help clear the abscess. I was totally amazed to find that nine hours after applying the poultice, all the pus had gone leaving only pink clean skin visible around the puncture hole in his head. Buzz was very definitive in his choices and the amounts he needed. Normally this type of wound would take 10 -12 days to heal.

Working in a cat rescue centre
Sam Davis, ex-zookeeper

Working in a cat rescue centre has provided lots of opportunities to collect data on cats and aromatic medicines. Obviously, if a cat is on veterinary medicines I am very limited in the use of essential oils. I have had some very alarming moments, for example, a cat sniffed an oil, choked then brought up a lot of phlegm. I've also had some very frustrating moments when I thought that nothing was working. However, most of the time, the experience has proved very rewarding and intriguing. Knowing that making even a small difference can have a dramatic effect on the lives of rescue animals is very rewarding. Cats come into our Sanctuary for a variety of reasons:

Strays: We have no information about these cats, what they have had to endure or how long they have been straying. 99.9% have no identification and probably about 35% have some kind of physical problem.

From homes: owners moving house / gone into a nursing home / passed away / cat not getting on with other pets , babies, children/ spraying / litter tray problems.

Not all cats from homes are in good condition! It should be remembered that most cats in the rescue centre are very stressed. This appears to heighten their emotions, increasing their need for oils. As yet, the majority of my studies have been done with rescue cats. It will be interesting to work with cats that are firmly established in a loving home environment and see what differences there are. What follows is an account of rescue cats that I have helped with aromatic medicines:

A long haired, tabby with a flea allergy

Charlotte was a lovely cat, but she wasn't too keen on other cats or children and preferred adult company. She was one of those cats with a great strength of character, which was just as well because a lot had happened in her life. Charlotte came to the centre because her owner was ill. Never have I seen such a neglected looking cat coming in from a home. Charlotte had a very bad flea allergy and her skin was in a terrible state with lots of open sores and scabs. She had had treatment for her fleas prior to coming in, strangely enough, she didn't seem to be in any discomfort.

I wanted to see the effects of chickweed macerated oil on the skin, as it is reputed to be very good. Charlotte was really keen and eagerly lapped up about 10 mls in one go. I offered her more throughout the day, and left some for the night staff to give her. Virtually overnight the sores started to dry up and the scabs loosened. Over the next 3 days Charlotte drank about 150 mls. and I am pleased to say that her stools weren't affected. By day four Charlotte had started to go off the chickweed and was only having a couple of licks.

When the vet next saw her she commented on how well her skin had healed and how her coat had improved, this was only 1 week later! I didn't say anything though because I would rather show the management what could be achieved using aromatic medicines before involving this particular vet that was very sceptical.

A 2 year old, female with a vaccine reaction

Magic was found as a stray with an injury to her back leg. The lady who found her kept her for a week, but her own cat wasn't happy about her arrival, so Magic came to us. She had a discharge from her eyes and was put on Aureomycin, an antibiotic eye cream. She also had a wound on her leg which was swollen and leaking pus, so she was given a 7 day course of antibiotics (Synulox). Her leg healed nicely and her eyes cleared up, then ten days later Magic had her first vaccination. This was followed by a clear discharge from her eyes, a slight discharge from her nose and sneezing. Apparently she had started sneezing the day after her vaccination.

I decided to offer her the following

Sandalwood	upper respiratory tract infections / conjunctivitis / skin disorders.
Frankincense	fear (encourages long slow deep breaths) / respiratory problems of an emotional origin / anti-catarrhal and expectorant properties
Lavender	gently relaxing / emotional disturbances manifested in the lungs / mild immune stimulant
Sea buckthorn	disorders of the skin and coat / lungs / proud flesh
Rosehip extract CO_2	cellular regeneration / immune stimulant / skin disorders
Seaweed	excellent for run-down animals / detoxifies / immune stimulant
Chickweed	soothing to skin / lubricates, soothes and protects internal mucous membranes

Day 1 - am

Magic inhaled the oils readily with much licking of the air. She wasn't overly keen on the seaweed but she eagerly consumed about 10 mls of chickweed. At noon I gave her more chickweed. The eye discharge lessened considerably and I only heard a couple of sneezes. The remedies were offered again at about 4pm and again she readily inhaled them, drinking more chickweed. The night staff also gave her more chickweed.

Days 2 & 3

The remedies were offered am and pm. Magic refused lavender, but showed a moderate interest in the rest. There were a few sneezes but no eye discharge, only discharge from the nose. More chickweed was taken.

Days 4 & 5

The remedies were offered once daily, and provoked only a slight interest. By day five everything was refused.

Days 6 - 9

Nothing was offered as I felt they were no longer needed. One big change I noticed was the quality of Magic's coat, it was incredibly soft with a lovely shine to it. The hair where the leg wound had been was also growing back very well.

Days 10 - 13

Magic was given her second vaccination today. By the afternoon she had started sneezing / snuffling again so I offered her the remedies. A moderate interest was shown in sandalwood, sea buckthorn and rosehip, but she did not want the chickweed. Magic preferred to take the oils late afternoon and by day 13 there was no more sneezing.

Days 14 & 15

No remedies offered. No more sneezing heard.

Day 16

We moved Magic over to the main cat section in the morning. Just as a precaution, I offered Magic her oils and she was interested in sandalwood and frankincense (interestingly oils for fear and comfort).

Days 17 & 18

Sandalwood and frankincense offered again but only very slight interest.

Notes

During her two week stay in the main cat area, Magic had the odd day where she would sneeze and snuffle. So I just offered her sniffs of her remedies to keep her topped up. I believe that Magic was a cat flu carrier and that the oils had kept her symptoms at bay. When Magic was homed she settled in very well with no recurrence of her sneezing or snuffling. Since Magic, I have had other cats with flu-like symptoms - sneezing, snuffling, leaky eyes and nasal discharge. The oils sandalwood, frankincense, lavender and the extracts sea buckthorn, rosehip and seaweed along with chickweed have proved very beneficial. I would not hesitate to bathe eyes with sandalwood if needed (provided the cat approved of course!) as I have used it successfully on my own cat. If a cat had a really blocked, runny nose I would steam bath first and maybe even put a drop or two of sandalwood in the steamer.

Depression: A 7 year old

Noelle's owners were moving into a flat and could not take her, so they found her a home living with a man who after two weeks rejected her as she wasn't a lap cat. Noelle then came to the rescue centre. She was a gentle cat who needed time to settle before she opened up. She didn't like children or other cats and was a lap cat, but only on her own terms and only with certain people. Noelle didn't like being picked up and was passed by because she spent most of her day curled up asleep in or under her bed. She became very depressed and had bouts of refusing to eat. The vet checked her over but could find nothing wrong, we were very worried about her. I had just finished the first part of the Animal Aromatics course and hoped that I could help. I had a limited amount of oils at that point but I thought about trying the following:

Rose otto	Past trauma / unwanted memories / anger / resentment / gladdens the heart
Lavender	Comforting / calming / relaxing / May help clear past habits and lessen irritability
Linden blossom	Physical and emotional abuse / lifts heavy emotions / relieves nervous tension
Marigold	works on a deeply emotional level and helps to comfort a sad heart
Lime flower	very calming / excellent for stress

Day 1
Noelle was under the bed when I went in. I offered her rose which she sniffed at intently, with lots of air licking and then came out towards the bottle. She started purring and slow blinking, this reaction was repeated with lavender essential oil. The strongest response, however was to the linden blossom, Noelle spent a long time with her nose right up against the bottle. She showed a slight interest in marigold and lime flower.

Day 2
Noelle came straight out from under the bed when I went in her pen. The rose offered a moderate interest with air licking and lots of purring but there was only slight interest in the lavender. Linden blossom was the favourite again, she inhaled this deeply from the bottle and became very relaxed. There was stronger interest in marigold compared with yesterday with deep inhalation and air licking. A slight interest was shown in lime flower.

Day 3
Noelle was in the top of the bed and jumped out when I entered. She was purring very loudly and rubbing all around my legs. She was slightly interested in the rose and linden blossom, had no interest in the lavender and a moderate interest in marigold and lime flower. I found it very difficult offering her the oils as she kept on head butting my hand and I didn't want to spill any oils on her. I have had this reaction quite a few times with cats, especially after offering them rose.

Day 4
Again very difficult to offer the oils as Noelle was being very affectionate and wouldn't leave me alone (not that I minded!)
Rose and lavender - no interest.
Linden blossom - moderate interest.
Marigold and lime flower - slight interest.

Day 5
No real interest in any of the oils but we did have a nice cuddle.

Notes
Noelle became more animated and actually showed more interest in the public, she was quite chatty at times. Three weeks later Noelle was homed to a lovely couple, who send us photos of her, in one she was being cuddled in the man's arms.

Sneezes and snuffles in the cattery

Just recently we had an outbreak of mild cat flu in the main cattery. Thankfully it was very mild with just sneezes and snuffles - no sore eyes, nasal discharge or cats going off their food. Usually if a cat starts sneezing we move it to the isolation block, but we had some newborn kittens in isolation and didn't want to risk infecting them. As the outbreak was so mild we decided that the cats would stay put. Two cats started off with sneezes and snuffles then seven more followed over the next few days. I thought that this was a good 'opportunity' to make a study, so chose three cats to offer 'respiratory' oils to.

Anneka: 4 years old
Spike: (the Magnificent): 12 years old
Peanut: 8 months old, ex-farm kitten with a grade 3 heart murmur.
Grommet: (Peanut's sister) was in the same pen, but never came down with any symptoms of cat flu.

I decided to offer oils that had in the past proven effective in the treatment of cat flu:

Frankincense	releases fears / encourages long, slow, deep breaths / indicated for lung problems of an emotional origin / possesses anti-catarrhal and expectorant properties
Sandalwood	good for upper respiratory tract infections as it has a pronounced action on the mucous membranes / skin problems / conjunctivitis / ear infections / comforts the body, mind and spirit while easing fears
Sea buckthorn	good for disorders of the lungs as it enhances the formation of tissues and antibodies general tonic / high vitamin C content
Rosehip extract	aids cellular regeneration / immune stimulant / high vitamin C content
Seaweed extract	immune stimulant / detoxifies / moistens dryness / soothes inflammations, packed with nutrients and minerals / great for run down, ageing animals

The oils were offered by self selection once a day only (due to time restrictions)

Anneka

She had started sneezing the day before, she sounded quite snuffly.
Frankincense - only slight interest.
Sandalwood - very strong interest. Came up to the bottle, lots of inhalation and air licking.
Sea buckthorn - very strong interest, came up to the bottle, lots of inhalation and air licking.
Rosehip extract CO_2 - very slight interest.
Seaweed extract - very strong interest, came up to the bottle and tried to lick the top. She obviously needed it so I put a drop on my finger - not that easy as the extract is very thick and difficult to get out of the bottle! Anneka licked my finger and wanted more. She took about four drops. I thought she might like to try some

kelp; I offered her a piece of the dried kelp which she took but spat it out immediately so I put some in her water bowl to soak. As Anneka sniffed at the bowl, I fished out a piece of soggy kelp and put it on her food mat. She ate it followed by a few more pieces and a few laps of the water. I put another water bowl down for her. Anneka continued to sneeze but not as often and was noticeably less snuffly.

Spike
Spike started sneezing two days after Anneka did. I was keen to include him in my study as he was an older cat and I did not want him to suffer too much.
Frankincense - immediately disappeared through the cat flap!
Sandalwood - strong interest, came up to the bottle and inhaled deeply with lots of air licking.
Sea buckthorn - strong interest, came up to the bottle and inhaled with lots of air licking.
Rosehip extract CO_2 - moderate interest, inhaled and air licked a few times.
Seaweed extract - similar reaction to rosehip. He showed no interest in soaked kelp.
As with Anneka after having his first lot of oils the sneezing had noticeably lessened.

Peanut
This was an amusing one and rather painful! Peanut probably sneezed the most out of the 3 cats. He was more snuffly with some clear discharge from his nose.
Frankincense - strong emotional release, lashed out at the bottle nearly knocking it from my hand (yep, he drew blood!).
Sandalwood - very deep inhalation and lots of air licking. Peanut purred very loudly and rubbed his head on my hand holding the bottle.
Sea buckthorn - moderate interest with air licking, purred again and rubbed his head on my hand.
Rosehip CO_2 - similar reaction to sea buckthorn.
Seaweed extract - lashed out at the bottle. I was ready this time and managed to avoid getting slashed. He showed no interest in soaked kelp.
Peanut was very specific in his responses. As with the other cats the sneezing had noticeably lessened after the first session with the oils. He did continue to sound very snuffly though, but there was no more clear discharge.

Summary
All three cats showed a definite preference for sandalwood and sea buckthorn. Both Anneka and Spike stopped sneezing / snuffling after 5 days. Peanut stopped sneezing / snuffling after 6 days.
The seven cats that were not offered any oils sneezed and snuffled for 10-15 days. It would be interesting to do a similar study with other respiratory oils such as lavender, myrrh, eucalyptus and lemon along with sandalwood and sea buckthorn to see if any, in particular, are preferred.

Urination problems
Rosie Wibberley 2004

Alfie moved to her present abode 3 months ago and had trouble settling in. She has been with her owner since she was a few weeks old and has moved over a dozen times in her life, but this is the first time she has found it difficult adjusting to her new surroundings. She moved from the city to a farm which is home to 6 other cats, which her owner felt frightened her. Alfie is normally a friendly, outgoing cat but she became withdrawn, spending a large amount of time under the bed, wanting to come in as soon as she was put outside. Uncharacteristically, she started urinating on the furniture, much to her owner's distress!

When I first met Alfie, she seemed friendly and immediately curious in the contents of my box. There was definitely something in their that she was interested in. I offered her cornflower water anyway, to open her up to healing, she showed no interest, so I then offered rose otto for possible emotional trauma or resentment in the change in circumstances. She showed a definite interest and licked her lips. I then offered violet leaf absolute, a popular remedy for animals that have recently moved, to comfort her heart and find her inner strength. Again she showed interest and licked her lips, but was not interested in taking either of these remedies orally. Chickweed macerated oil was then offered which she tentatively licked from my fingers. Chickweed is a remedy often selected by cats and is an adaptogen. We then offered her neroli for sadness and separation but she just gave me a look as if to say 'that's not what I need' and walked away! We tried offering jasmine absolute, to ease her nervousness and hopefully eradicate the problem of urinating in the house, which she showed a slight interest in, and also in Roman chamomile, which was also offered to ease her nerves. We then spread rose petals, lime flowers, arnica flowers and chickweed herb into small heaps. Alfie liked sitting on the rose petals, but showed no interest in any of the others.

There was however, definitely still something in my box that she was interested in, and without too much ado, she inhaled spirulina from the bag, but showed no interest in taking it internally. She also appeared to be interested in green clay, which she licked from her owner's fingers. We then offered seaweed extract to her which she sniffed at the bottle several times before yawning and licking her lips. It turned out that Alfie was born near the sea and spent the first few years of her life within 200 yards of the coast, so there may have been some association with the seaweed. Seaweed offers an abundance of nutrients and can be useful for detoxification. I left some seaweed extract, green clay and macerated chickweed for Alfie.

The evening after I saw Alfie, she sat on the beanbag at her owners feet and made a huge puddle! I was mortified. I thought that maybe the oils hadn't helped at all. However, the next day, she ventured out into the yard for the first time and over the following weeks she started going out more regularly, after two weeks she was asking to be let out and venturing further afield. She has stopped urinating in the house (since that final incident with the bean bag!). She regularly (every 2 or 3 days) sniffs the seaweed extract, but hasn't been interested in anything else.

Rodents & rabbits
Guinea pigs, chinchillas, degus, rabbits

As with all captive animals it is important to study how caged animals such as guinea pigs, chinchillas and hamsters behave and live in their natural habitat, in order to make their life more comfortable. For example, Guinea pigs which, originated from South America, live in large family groups, being protected from predators by the overhanging stems of the long grasses that they make their home in. Even though they don't burrow for themselves they use abandoned burrows from other animals.

In their environment they bathe, not in water but in clay or dry sandy soil, it is not unusual for them to also roll their food in clay. So if you want to make your rodent feel more comfortable and 'at home' try offering powdered green clay in a tray or large dish. This also works as a flea powder.

Don't forget when leaving aromatics in the cage make sure that animals can escape from the aromas.

These herbivores will generally prefer the essential oils and the dried remedies to macerated oils. Devil's claw, rosehips and spirulina are popular. Preferred oils can be left on a rag, in water or on grass.

A 'tail' of two Degus
Sarah Kinson and Debbie Green 2003 In class at the Ingraham school

Degus are naturally diabetic, they lack the ability to digest sugar in their food. Even the sugars in an apple can lead to eventual death. Never try to catch a degu by his tail, in defence against their natural enemies, degus can lose the end of their tails. The result is a bloody injury, and the end of their tail never grows back again. If left untreated, a degloved tail can get infected. If degus feel threatened or uncomfortable, they usually make a loud 'weep' noise.

The teeth of a healthy degu are yellow or orange, white teeth are an indication of a serious disease. Degus' teeth become orange a couple of weeks after their birth, due to a reaction from the chlorophyll from green plants with the degus' saliva. Degus are sociable animals, so it is best to keep at least two. A degu, will not be happy on its own and will not live as long as with a companion. If kept alone, it could become depressed and it may cause it to become aggressive. As degus are social animals they rarely bite a person or another degu.

Degus originate from the West Coast of Chile to the Andes Mountains where, they live in large groups, making their homes in rocks or brush.
The pair we were working with were brought to the rescue centre the day before we arrived. They were hiding in their wooden house, burrowed in amongst fresh newspaper cuttings. They had not come out since their arrival and had apparently been making 'weeping noises' during this time. Our first challenge was to encourage them from their hiding hole without forcibly removing them and scaring them further. Caroline had some fresh celery sticks in her kit and these proved invaluable. No one was keen to offer fingers to sharp toothed Degus who may be feeling threatened and scared.

We started with angelica root, holding the bottle close to the entrance of their home. There was some promising rustling, but nothing further. We tried rose otto and got no response. After about half an hour of repeatedly offering the two oils Caroline suggested we try spirulina, by putting some in a bowl outside their house. There was again a promising rustle, but still no degu. So we covered the end of the celery stick in Spirulina, then Caroline gently eased it into their hiding place; almost immediately out popped the braver of the two. Initially he ran around making 'weep' noises, but soon quietened down and was quite happy to sniff some rose otto also applied to the end of a celery stick. We then tried a drop of rosehip extract using the same method; this sent the little degu into a trance-like state for some minutes.

In the Degu's natural habitat they would bath and roll in areas of their terrain; so we put some rough green clay in a shallow bowl. A short while later when he discovered the 'clay' bath, and it was with great gusto (and probably relief) that he bathed and groomed himself in it many times during that afternoon. He also ran in the spirulina and then straight into the clay, mixing the two in his bowl. Later he appeared to purposely drop his food into the bowl of clay, then picked it out again and ate it, with a light dusting of clay mixed with spirulina.

We then began to work with the other degu, which was still hiding in her wooden house, so we put a drop of frankincense (for fear) onto another trusty celery stick and introduced it to her. There was a rustle and then she ate the part of the celery that was laced with the frankincense, after which she became very still; seconds later she popped out of her house, and then went quickly back inside to re-emerge a few seconds later. We then tried rose otto and rosehip with the same results. Rosehip sent the degu off into a dreamy state which lasted a couple of minutes. After a good 'bath' in the green clay, they groomed each other thoroughly, playing happily together. After that day there was no turning back and these two degus developed a social interactive relationship with their carers.

A guinea pig with skin problems
Donna Scotter

Len is a four month old ginger and black, short-haired guinea pig who has been with his owners since he was eight weeks old. He appeared to be in good health except for a problem with his skin which was dry, flaky and scabby in areas where it had been bleeding. As a result his owners had not been able to pick him up for some time as when they did he squealed as if in pain and he would try to bite them. They couldn't think of any changes they had made that might have triggered an allergic reaction. When Len was offered oils he hid in the corner of his cage.

Len was being fed on guinea pig food, apple bars and carrots. I advised his owners to stop feeding him apple bars as they have a high sugar content and are made for human consumption.

Based on his history and his condition, I left German chamomile and neroli; both diluted in water, they were put in water bowls in his cage separate from his usual water supply. I also made a spray using hydrolats (floral waters) of Roman chamomile, lavender and tea tree. Len did not obviously go to the water bowls but would have inhaled trace amounts in the cage, however, he seemed to enjoy being sprayed. A week after starting his remedies Len had no open sores and all the scabs had healed. One month later his skin had completely recovered and the fur had grown back.

In this case it is unclear if the positive outcome is a result of the remedies, cutting out the apple bars or a mixture of both.

A Chinchilla: not his usual self
Penny Ward 2006

Charlie was to be taken to the vets at the weekend due to behavioural changes. He didn't run around as much when he was let out of his cage and when he did, he didn't kick his back heels up like he usually did. There was a feeling that generally Charlie wasn't the cheerful chinchilla that he used to be. I read up as much as possible on chinchilla's; including their natural habitat and diet. They originated from the Andes where it is very cold and they are naturally nocturnal animals, which mainly forage on grasses. I arranged to go and see Charlie, but felt slightly nervous as he would be my first 'proper' case study and I had no experience of working with chinchillas.

Charlie has been with his present owner for about five months and is about four years old. His previous owners had kept him in a tiny bird cage where he was not often allowed out. He now has a large cage with shelves fitted for him to jump around on. His owner explained that they had recently moved house, to a new house, one which is a lot warmer. This coupled with the fact that his cage is also situated next to a radiator, means that he is most likely extremely warm. The Andes is cold and chinchillas have thick coats. It was mentioned that when Charlie comes out of his cage he runs to the back of a table, by a wall under the window. I immediately thought this was perhaps to cool down.

When I first entered the room and put the boxes of oils on the floor Charlie ran over and sat on them. I took the lids of selected oils (for anxiety and fear) and put the bottles on the floor scattered around the room; we left Charlie alone with them while we observed him. The oils included rose absolute, yarrow, neroli, bergamot, frankincense, and Roman chamomile. He ran around the room for a while before approaching the essential oil bottles. He went straight to rose absolute, and sat with his nose just above the bottle top, inhaling. Charlie didn't approach the yarrow at all, but he licked the top of the bergamot and neroli bottle and inhaled and licked the Roman chamomile and the frankincense bottle.

All this took place over about 20 minutes to half an hour. After a while Charlie took himself back into his cage to rest, he looked so relaxed and as if he was processing the oils. We left him for a while and after some time and discussion we decided to offer him ylang ylang for self worth and confidence. When he was in his cage, we needed to hold the bottle from the outside in order to offer it to him, as he would not normally be happy for anyone to put their hand in his cage, but as I opened the bottle of ylang ylang Charlie ventured forward to the aroma, I decided to put my hand in the cage and he put his front claws onto the bottle as he inhaled the oil. He was transfixed to this oil, taking in large, deep inhalations, he did not move away for a least a minute. His owner was amazed that he was accepting a hand in his cage! We continued to observe Charlie who again appeared very quiet, relaxed and peaceful.

After letting him rest we reoffered him all of the oils; the ones he was most keen on were

> Roman chamomile - anxiety
> Frankincense - fear
> Bergamot - balancing
> Ylang ylang - self worth/confidence

I made up dilutions in water and left them for Charlie. It was decided that he would be offered the oils every evening. I advised that if he licked the bottle to pour the oil onto the finger tip so he could take it orally if he wanted, and to let him inhale the oil for as long as he wanted until he moved away, giving him time to process any information he was obtaining from the oil.

Results

Charlie selected the oils for 30 days, some days licking some days inhaling. Charlie's owner commented throughout this time that he was becoming more relaxed and seemed much happier in his surroundings. She felt that Charlie enjoyed the time that was set aside for him to take his remedies and that the process had a bonding effect between the chinchilla, herself and her partner who often offered the remedies.

I revisited Charlie about two months later and was amazed at the change in his temperament. He was not at all withdrawn and when his owner opened the cage he literally jumped into her arms. When he was put on the floor he came running up to me (more or less a stranger to him) for attention; he looked brighter in himself and more confident. He also kicks up his heels again when he runs about, something that he had stopped doing before his oils. His cage has been enlarged and moved away from the radiator to the cooler side of the room and he now has a new mate Marble, a female chinchilla.

Authors note: It may have been interesting to observe his reaction to peppermint oil (cooling), which was not offered at the time.

Avian

Birds generally select essential oils for inhalation and dried remedies such as rosehips and spirulina orally. The health of birds especially chicken can be transformed with spirulina, including the laying of healthy eggs; the results can be astonishing. Another remedy that offers impressive results for a poorly chicken is watered down honey.

Powdered remedies such as spirulina should be offered as a watery paste, in water or dry. Essential oils can be left in individual water bowls, large enough to dunk their head in - which they frequently do!

A pheasant at Sparsholt College, Winchester showed a spectacular response after the inhalation of pink lotus oil. He gave a full display of his feathers, something that had never been seen before in all the time he has been at the college, which is in excess of two years. To everyone's astonishment the pheasant didn't attack the man offering the bottle, (he usually gets quite aggressive towards men), whom he had attacked the previous day when he was working in his enclosure.

A parrot constantly screaming for attention
Elizabeth Soames

Peefer, a conure parrot constantly screams for attention, is possessive of his owner Andy and shows aggressive behaviour especially around his cage area.

Peefer recently had quite a few changes in his life, he had moved home from a flat which was very quiet, to a house where the neighbours could be heard, as well as having another person and a puppy to share his new house with. He was no longer the centre of attention and was finding it hard to share. Due to his constant screaming he had to move from sitting by the patio door up to the office where it was quieter and where the neighbours could not wind him up once he started screaming.

Background
Peefer was captive bred and then placed into a pet shop aviary at a young age, he was chosen because he was the small, runty one with a battered tail who had obviously been picked on.

Parrots are naturally very nervous birds - they are normally alert and wary of everything going on in their environment. In the wild conures tend to do everything in a group with parrots of the same breed; this gives the birds the security that they need. Within the group they build up an order where the younger and less confident birds follow the example of the leaders. From the leaders they take the cue when to flee or hide from predators, where to feed and where to sleep.

For captive bred birds the security of the flock is not available and they may look to their owner to give them guidance. Most of the birds are removed from their parents when they are still inside the egg and then hand reared. The lack of contact and learning from their own kind can lead to behavioural problems and can make them vulnerable to psychological problems.

Treatment

The remedies selected were neroli, ylang ylang, vetiver, xantham gum, devil's claw and chalk. The oils were offered in the above order and devils claw, xantham gum and chalk were placed in his cage so that he could help himself ad lib.

To start with I offered Peefer each oil individually while he was out of his cage so that he could get away from the aroma if he chose to. He was offered neroli which could help him with any feelings of loss or sadness linked to his early months of hand rearing and being on his own in the pet shop where he missed out on essential contact and learning from his parents. When offered neroli he moved around eyeing up the bottle. After a short while he came up and touched the bottle with his beak, he then backed off and pretended to be busy doing other things, rubbing his beak, picking up seeds or having a drink but all the time he was keeping an eye on the bottle, which he then came back to, touched again and backed off before losing interest.

Ylang ylang was offered next. This could help him with lack of confidence and is comforting. These are feelings he would have naturally got from being in a flock and having leaders to look up to and guide him. When he was offered the ylang ylang, he came straight up to it, inhaled the aroma for quite some time and then tried to get hold of the bottle with his beak. I re-offered it again after a few minutes break, and he gave the same response, so I put 3 drops into a small bowl of water and placed it in the holder inside his cage.

Peefer is usually very wary of something new in his environment, but he came straight over, licked the bowl, walked away, then come back to it almost immediately and dunked his head into the ylang ylang water. Shaking off the excess, he then repeated this behaviour, drinking some of the water along with fresh water. He did this for about 5 minutes before he lost interest. He then went to the back of his cage and perched as he does when he rests. I decided to give him a break at this stage and offer his other remedies the next day.

Vetiver helps with 'grounding' and can give a sense of belonging. When Peefer was offered vetiver he puffed up his feathers and tried to peck at the bottle, becoming very still he breathed the aroma in slowly. Peefer stayed close to the bottle for a few minutes before moving away to eat. In between seeds he came back for more and eventually licked the bottle before moving away and losing interest.

Devil's claw, xantham gum and chalk were all offered and selected, they must have contained a supplement or property that he needed - he has no supplements in his diet and has never taken to cuttle fish for calcium. This could be why he wanted chalk and maybe he selected devil's claw as he was in some sort of pain or discomfort of which we were not aware.

Devil's claw was offered through the bars of his cage. He came straight to it and started to peck at it (this was unusual as normally he is cautious of new things). A few slices were put into a bowl in his cage so he could help himself, he picked pieces up and had a good peck and chew, making sure he didn't drop any of it, which was surprising as parrots are naturally wasteful, dropping their food to just go and get more. He has continued to have devil's claw ad lib daily.

When he was offered xantham gum he rushed over and took a large mouthful without checking what it was first, he then came back for the rest of it. For the next few days he got very excited every time the packet was opened and his bowl topped up. Peefer was slightly more cautious when he was offered chalk. He had a good look and smell of it first before taking a good sized mouthful, he then shook his head and came back for more. He has the chalk ad lib along with xantham gum and devil's claw. Peefer has his oils offered once a day as he has not been interested in taking them more frequently.

Behavioural changes

After approximately one week Peefer's aggression was greatly reduced. People other than Andy could safely put food through the bars without risk of being bitten, his screaming reduced and didn't continue for as long (mainly only when the toilet was flushed in the morning). He became chattier, greeting people with a hello and a chirrup instead of backing away or screaming. He now was spending more time at the front of his cage, asking for more cuddles and allowing more contact with different people.

Two weeks after Peefer took his initial remedies

People could easily put their fingers into the cage without risk of being bitten. His plumage changed - even though it looked good before the colours were more vibrant. He was much more interactive and vocal in a gentle communicative way, making quieter more contented noises. He generally seemed happier within himself and more confident in his surroundings.

Six weeks after Peefer took his initial remedies

His behaviour has greatly improved, his confidence has grown and he is more relaxed. He is happy with his cage door open for long periods of time and his screaming has greatly reduced (normally only when you haven't been in to see him in the morning). When he is out of his cage he is much more inquisitive and has the confidence to explore instead of staying within close proximity of the cage. He doesn't panic as easily, for example, his cage cover fell on him and he just shook it off and walked away - the old Peefer would have panicked and screamed.

Peefer is still offered his oils on a regular basis but he picks and chooses which one he wants on which day, he still wants xantham gum and chalk but he doesn't have devil's claw as often.

Farm animals

Goats and rams

My experience of working with goats is that they will always make it very obvious that they want their remedy applied to their head and horns. Other than by inhalation, this is often their preferred application.

A ram that I worked with was so aggressive, no one other than the keeper at the rare breeds centre, was allowed to enter the enclosure. The ram was to be destroyed as he was a danger to anyone who may wander in to his paddock - the rams focus was to attack.

I offered (through the fence!) rose otto to which he licked the air, neroli which caused fast shallow breathing and yarrow which stimulated a strong emotional release, on inhalation he head butted the fence just missing my hand! He then ate six slices of devil's claw and drank and ate soaked seaweed. Shortly after the ram took the remedies, the keeper walked into the enclosure with the rose otto on his hand, he walked up to the ram, who for the first time in two years did not make an attempt to charge. The onlookers were amazed with what they saw as the keeper knelt down beside him, gently massaging the rams head with his rose covered hand. The keeper and ram then walked away from each other in peace. This was televised on a Channel 4 documentary 2003. 'Talking to Animals'.

An Aggressive goat
Leigh Smith 2004

Daisy is a six year old Angora x Pygmy goat. I was told she was aggressive and bad tempered, her owner joked that she would not go anywhere near her. Daisy has been at her present home since she was two, little is known of her past, except that she may have had a kid before coming to live there. Daisy lives with the horses on the livery yard and has her own stable. She eats their same feed, grazes and eats bark where she can. Physically she is well, but the main concern is that she has difficulty coping with children, strangers and most of all the owners' mother, who she will head butt when ever she possibly can. For this reason she is kept tethered except when the owner is in the yard.

I offered Daisy oils to help with past traumas and mental stimulation, while doing so I asked the owner to hold the tether in case the goat decided to head butt me. I wanted to give off signals of calm, not fear, but as it happened, I need not have had any concerns because throughout the whole session Daisy was calm and relaxed with me, lowering her head to the floor, not pulling on the tether once. She was very interested in the oils.

I offered her: angelica seed and root, rose otto and absolute, neroli, linden blossom, vetiver, vanilla, valerian, bergamot, ylang ylang, violet leaf, peppermint and spearmint. I also offered devil's claw but she was only interest in eating the paper bag it was in (proving they will not eat these secondary compounds if they are not needed). The oils that she was most interested in were bergamot, ylang ylang and spearmint. With these three oils Daisy lowered her head, positioning it so that my hand holding the bottle was made to rub the area between her horns, then up her horns. She was very much in control of this process and seemed calm and content to have her head so low. Until now, she had never been seen to flehmen, go into a trance, or rub her head and horns on anything held out to her. Her owner and others watching were also amazed how calm she was in my presence, not attempting to injure me, much to my own relief too!

The oils were diluted into a sunflower base and offered once or twice a day depending on her needs. I asked them to follow the principles of self selection and that they should take Rosie's lead on the use of the oils.

Results

Throughout the first two weeks of using the oils, Daisy continued in much the same way; lowering her head to have them rubbed on her brow and horns, appearing very calm and relaxed, occasionally showing the flehmen response to ylang ylang. She continued with this interest for a further week before it lessened, by the end of week three she no longer wanted the oils.

According to her owner Daisy is so much more relaxed with everyone, although she does still chase the owner's mother! So I recommended that any future offering of oils should be done by the owner's mother in order to develop a bond between them.

Lambs with E. coli & my husband
By Dida Wales 2006

We try to plan lambing so it falls on Easter weekend. This year, between Easter Sunday and the following Thursday morning our ewes had produced 15 healthy lambs. Unfortunately by Thursday afternoon my husband Mark was feeling extremely unwell, so came home from work early. By the time I returned at around 7 pm, he had a very high temperature, diarrhoea, violent sickness and a pounding headache. He wasn't in a good state. Mark was getting worse as the evening went on, in desperation I looked through some clinical human aromatherapy books, and found a reference to cinnamon bark essential oil in one of Kurt Schnaubelt's publications. It stated that cinnamon bark oil was antibacterial, antifungal, antiviral, safe for internal use and particularly useful for stomach upsets.

I was a bit wary of using an ill husband as a trial but Mark was almost hallucinating (he gets a bit dramatic), crying out and balled up in pain, so I thought - what the hell…! I put 2 drops of the oil into a pint of water, which he sipped at gingerly. After pulling lots of faces at the thought, he said it didn't taste too bad and managed a good inch of water before laying back in bed. Within two minutes he was quiet, and within ten minutes he was asleep - fantastic. He woke a few times in the night and managed to keep sipping the cinnamon bark water. By the morning he had drunk half a pint and was absolutely fine - by 2 pm that afternoon he was brick laying!

During this time of course, while I was keeping an eye on the new lambs, and I noticed that one of the youngest was looking a bit dehydrated.

Unfortunately upon examination, it was clear that the lamb had diarrhoea, and was quite poorly, so I popped it into the lambing pen with its mother and took its temperature - very high. Like all new born animals this can be pretty serious and I was concerned; I tried to bottle feed the lamb with electrolytes but by this stage it was too weak and required stomach tube feeding. I did this and then left the lamb for half an hour to rest in the pen with its mother. When I checked on the lamb again her temperature had dropped dramatically, but she was still in a feverish state, so she came into the advanced lamb hospital we have - a cardboard box in the sitting room.

At this time we also noticed that other lambs in the flock had also developed diarrhoea and were looking very drawn. It was obvious they too were suffering from an infection such as E. coli or campylobacter; both these bugs can easily take the life of a young lamb. Before I called in the vet I thought I would try the cinnamon bark that Mark had taken 24 hours earlier. Little Paula in the lamb hospital was too weak to indicate if she wanted the oil, but the other lambs that were just coming down with the illness were interested in its aroma and inhaled a little, so we made up fresh bottles of lamb-aid (electrolytes with calcium and magnesium) with 60 ml of water and 1 drop of cinnamon bark essential oil. I also put 2 drops into a bucket of water for the lambs and ewes to select themselves if they wanted. We were able to offer the bottles regularly and with 15 lambs all poorly we spent most of the weekend chasing them. Paula was up by the next morning so we reunited her back with mum. By Saturday evening all lambs were showing a huge improvement and none were looking seriously ill anymore. The buckets that were put out for the girls to self - select had all been successful, this included individual buckets of rosehips, green clay, seaweed, plain water and cinnamon water. Paula still had a runny tum so we added green powdered clay to the water, which worked a treat. By Sunday morning the lambs no longer required the remedies in their bottles, but we continued to provide the buckets with extracts, they just loved the rosehips and green clay. I needed to re-fill each container twice a day just to keep up with them!

On the Monday we took Paula into our veterinary practice to identify the bug, which was diagnosed as E. coli. Normally an antibiotic, combined with clay and electrolytes would have been administered but the vet recommended us to continue as we were.

12 month old Dexter Heifer deglove injury to Horn
Victoria Morley 2006

We found Bramble Rose in the field with the outer horny layer to her horn missing and the horn stump bleeding profusely, so we put her in the cattle crush and placed a tourniquet on the horn bud, which slowed the bleeding a little, in that it was not running into her eye.

While in the crush I offered her the following: yarrow, carrot seed, lavender, rose otto and tea tree essential oil, arnica oil macerated oil and green clay. She tried to lick the yarrow and carrot seed but there was no response to the other remedies, other than rose which she inhaled, this seemed to have a calming effect on her, as she then stood calmly in the crush while I applied the paste to the horn.

The paste
2 tblsp powdered green clay, with just enough water to make it mouldable, but not too sloppy that it would run off the horn.
4 drops of yarrow and 4 drops of carrot seed.

At first the green clay paste looked wet but after a few moments it seemed to lose its moisture as though the horn was absorbing in the moisture and sealing itself. The wound did at this point stop bleeding. The vet was coming to see our cattle, the day after and this heifer was to be dehorned, but as the bleeding had stopped we decided that she would be alright to wait until the morning to see him.

A lamb with flystrike
Maxime Stewart 2006

Flystrike is where flies lay eggs on the fleece, these then hatch as maggots, which then burrow into the fleece. This is common to sheep with diarrhoea as the fleece becomes dirty, causing sores on the skin to become infected allowing the maggots to then burrow into the wounds.

Sadly with this particular lamb its mother was found dead in the field, during some very hot weather and the carcass was not found until the next day. As the carcass was infested with maggots, it was thought that the lamb had become infested too, from laying next to her.

When I first saw the lamb the wounds were quite extensive, the fleece had been clipped from around the back end, but the farmer had decided that the only option was to put it down, as the wounds were not healing. I asked if he would give me 48 hours to work with the lamb and if there was no improvement then I would leave its future up to him. He reluctantly agreed (mumbling under his breath that it was a waste of my time but if that was what I wanted!).

My first priority was to clear the maggots and to keep the flies away to prevent re-infestation. I cleaned the wound using 10 drops of tea tree in 1litre of warm water. Then I decided to try and protect the wound by covering it with green clay and aloe paste, which would also be used to suspend the oils in.

To determine which remedies were needed, I offered the following oils and noted the lamb's response.

Yarrow	Inhaled, mouthed but did not take any off the hand
Tea tree	Inhaled
Thyme thymol	Inhaled, mouthed
Yarrow	Inhaled, mouthed
German chamomile	Inhaled
Garlic	Inhaled, mouthed but did not take orally
Lavender	Inhaled, eyes closed
Sandalwood	No interest
Sea buckthorn	No interest

For behavioural trauma

Neroli	Not interested
Frankincense	Inhaled, eyes closed, quiet
Rose otto	Inhaled, eyes closed, quiet

The lamb showed interest in the following oils so I put them into a clay / aloe gel paste:

Clay paste

Lavender	10 drops
Tea tree	10 drops
Yarrow	7 drops
Thyme thymol	5 drops
Garlic	5 drops
German Chamomile	7 drops

Made up into 75ml clay paste

Fly spray Tabs

I also made up a spray for the surrounding area, to prevent further fly eggs being laid, this consisted of:

Lavender	10 drops
Tea tree	10 drops
Garlic	8 drops

Let down in aloe gel and water to make up to 200ml spray

After 3 days:

The infected area appeared to be shrinking and become more localised, the surrounding skin had died off leaving pink, healthy skin underneath. I later decided to add marigold macerated oil and sandalwood to the clay paste, to stop the skin drying out as much (the sandalwood was offered to her again and this time she responded positively, inhaling and licking).

After 6 days

One small area remained infected, however the surrounding tissue looked healthy, I made up a new aloe gel as the lamb was no longer interested in thyme and garlic.

Lavender	10 drops
Tea tree	7 drops
Yarrow	7 drops
Sandalwood	5 drops

in 75 mls of aloe vera gel

The above preparation was applied once a day for seven days, after which time the wound had completely healed. The lamb was put back into the flock with no further problems.

Exotics

The study on orang-utans demonstrates how primates treat themselves innately. So many people are subject to writing about the do's and don'ts of using essential oils. The orang-utans, however show us that it is possible to use instinctive knowing as a guide. I therefore consider this an important study to publish.

Orang-utans

Frances Fitzgerald Cleveland USA 2001

The first time we offered the orang-utans their essential oils we placed a few drops on a clean rag (each oil had its own rag), then we handed the rag to the orang-utans. If they liked it they would sniff it for long periods of time, or lick the rag. When Sally, one of the female orang-utans, really liked an oil she would place the rag with the oil on it into her mouth, fill her mouth up with water and proceed to suck the oil out of the rag - it was fascinating. If they did not like the oil they would hand us the rag back. One night Sally gathered all her favourite rags and placed them in her nest and slept with them. I thought of using the rags because I was afraid they would try to snatch the bottles out of our hands. The head zoo keeper thought as an initial approach, it was a great idea.

After a few days of working with the oils and the orang-utans, the zoo keepers were comfortable with the process and just showed them the oils bottle by bottle. This proved to work quite well except they had to be extra careful with Mias, as he grabbed a bottle once, pulled out the plunger, drank the contents and handed the bottle back as if asking for more. All of the orang-utans were very responsive to the process. They would smell the oil and then hold out their finger for some drops to be applied which, they would ether lick off or apply to their forehead, chest, arms or nose. Sometimes they would stick their chests out and want it rubbed in. Or they would stick their lips out and want it applied there. They were very clear on what oil they wanted and where they wanted it. If they were not interested in the oil they would turn their heads away or walk away.

The gorillas were completely different. When we went to hand them a rag with an oil on it they appeared insulted and would not even touch the rag, so we had to improvise here. I suggested we take some of their food pellets and apply the oils to them. This worked perfectly, if they did not like the oil they would throw the pellet of food back at us, if they liked the oils they would either ingest the pellet, or keep it to smell. When we worked with Koundo, the largest silver back gorilla in captivity, he was not impressed with the pellets, so I asked what his favourite snack was and his was leaves. We applied some oil to a leaf and if he liked it he would eat it, sniff it, or place it next to him. If he did not like it he handed it back. Later on the zoo keeper also worked with the bottles of oils, unless it was an aggressive gorilla and then she would use the food.

Robin, a 26 year old, male orang-utan

The problem the zoo keeper wanted to address with Robin, is that he became sexually aroused with human females, causing him to be rough with Sally (his mate). He would drag her around and forcefully copulate with her. Female visitors or female keepers that are not regularly in his building trigger this behaviour. Robin initially selected: jasmine, melissa, frankincense, vetiver, rose otto, vanilla, rosemary and geranium.

Two months later he selected: jasmine, melissa, frankincense, vetiver, rose otto, basil, sweet marjoram, angelica root and grapefruit. Robin is having success with the oils, and he has calmed down a great deal. He sometimes gets excited and chases after Sally, but these episodes are very infrequent now. The zoo keeper is pleased with the progress Robin is making.

Allie, a 7 year old, female orang-utan

Allie lost her mother just over a year ago, and then became seriously ill 3 months after her mother died. She underwent many tests and observations by vets, and became to distrust unfamiliar humans, whereas before her illness she loved everybody. What the zoo keeper wanted to accomplish with Allie and the oils, was to regain her trust of humans and bring her old personality back. I also felt she needed her immune system boosted. Oils selected: rose, yarrow, bergamot and melissa.

Allie has had great success with her oils. Many people have commented on how she seems like her old self as she is now once again playful and not depressed. Her zoo keeper is very pleased with the results.

Tigers
Article 'Your Cat' Magazine: February 2006

A solution was needed for a tiger who at times, was risking her own safety and that of her keepers. But who would have thought that her life would have been turned around by scent? The success achieved by aromatherapy pioneer Caroline Ingraham in introducing a sense of calm to a fearful tiger could offer hope for other big cats in captivity, not to mention domestic cats with issues!

Ronja is a three-and-a-half-year-old Siberian Tiger who was imported from Germany to the Wildlife Heritage Foundation in Kent two years ago. From her arrival she showed extreme rage towards men. Her attacks were so fierce that she would hurt herself and damage the fence at which she was hurling herself. Caroline says: "She became known within the zoo and exotic animal community as one of the most aggressive tigers they had ever known." Looking after her was not easy. It was impossible to shut her into her house when her enclosure was due to be cleaned, instead the neighbouring tiger was shut into his house and she was ushered into his enclosure. If ever she was shut in her house she became so violent that staff were afraid she would seriously hurt herself. Caroline adds: "It was at the point whereby they needed to decide if it was fair and safe to keep Ronja alive."

WHF Director Mark Edgerly invited Caroline over in August 2006. Although intrigued by the possibilities of what could be achieved using essential oils, Mark admits that he had initially been rather sceptical. Caroline's first step was to put undiluted drops of five chosen essential oils and one fixed oil on six-inch strips of plywood.

Here's what was selected

Linden blossom	physical injury/dislike of men, no interest
Rose otto	past trauma, - slight interest
Ylang Ylang	lack of self-worth/confidence - no interest
Vetiver	offers stability, slight interest
Frankincense	fear - frequently selected
Hemp oil	interested
Frankincense	fear - interested
Valerian	deep sedative - interested
Angelica root	opens the animal up to healing - interested
Sandalwood	fear / supports the kidneys, a weak area for both big and domestic cats: a very - strong interest
Peppermint	stimulant - interested

Caroline notes:
"She would walk a few steps away then return for more. She did this many times over a period of an hour." Hemp oil, which is calming to the central nervous system, she approached and licked.

Caroline explains: "When Ronja selects her remedy she will walk to the chosen plank of wood, circle it to lift the aroma and as she almost completes her circle she will grimace to draw it in." There was a stunning immediate result. "She walked into her house to retrieve her food while two men were stood by, something she had never done before." Five days later, the positive changes were apparent. Caroline recalls: 'As I stood by Ronja's enclosure she walked close to Mark, her keeper and director of WHF; he had never been so close to her before without being the subject of attack."

Caroline has since tried other oils, chosen to match Ronja's temperament and her habitat and allowed the tiger to select her favourites.

Caroline takes up the story: "Ronja walked straight to the Sandalwood. This oil prompted the strongest interest of all the oils to date, she returned to it many times over a period of two hours, displaying the flehmen response each time she inhaled its aroma. Ronja paraded up and down the side of the enclosure where the oils were placed, each time returning to the sandalwood, circling it and taking up the aroma. After about half an hour into the sandalwood selection she walked over to the peppermint, put her head down and inhaled it, going back to it several times. She also selected angelica root, which she returned to a number of times, while still intermittently selecting her sandalwood to which she was very attracted.

Eventually Ronja returned to her "comfort patch." Soon after Caroline had finished, a group of photographers arrived, part of a regular arrangement. Ronja's usual reaction was to go for the attack or more usually hide in her house. As she did the latter, Mark decided to see if the essential oil inhalation would have positive results allowing her to be shut in. To Mark's amazement she did! The house is designed so that the keepers can walk in and be protected by wire fencing.

At the first sign of the door opening in the past, Ronja would throw her entire body weight at the fencing by the keeper's door, which was distressing and dangerous for both the keeper and Ronja. "Mark went to the door, opening it slowly. Instead of throwing herself at the fence, Ronja lay in her bed, growling. As he took steps in, the growls turned to loud roars, however she still remained in her bed." The next experiment was for Mark to wear Ronja's favourite oils so that she would see him as a positive experience. "Rose had previously been selected but was not one of her favourites at the time, however from past experience I have observed that rose can help animals cope with stress," Caroline explains, so, rose was applied to Mark's chest, sandalwood to an arm and angelica root and frankincense on the other arm.

This time the effect was quite startling; Ronja allowed Mark to walk in, giving only the odd growl. He was able to sit down cross-legged in front of her (a wire fence separating them), while she closed an eye. He stayed there for a good ten minutes. That was the closest she had been to anyone in the time they had known her, something they had only experienced when she was anaesthetised. Mark says: "I went into the corridor expecting her to rant and rave like she used to, but she didn't. She curled up and put her head between her paws. I was just amazed!"

Since Caroline began to visit, Ronja has not attempted to attack men as violently as she did in the past and she is no longer considered a danger.

Since October, Ronja has even allowed herself to be shut in the house without a fuss. says Mark. Zoo professionals who saw her a year ago say they have noticed a remarkable difference in her. We don't experience the rages that we used to get. "Sandalwood is still her favourite, she will even take strips of wood with the oils on to the area of her enclosure where she eats." As far as Mark knows, she is the only big cat to experience the benefits of essential oils. He hopes that the success they are having will help others like her.

Ronja is a Siberian tiger, an endangered species. One year after working with her she is now in the breeding program - something that was thought to be out of the question

Nutrition

by Nick Thompson BSc (Hons), BVM&S, VetMFHom, MRCVS

Canine nutrition

Human nutrition is undergoing a revolution. On one side we are seeing increases in Irritable Bowel Syndrome (IBS), allergies, cancers and food intolerances. On the other, greater awareness of the role of nutrition as the foundation of all these human conditions is making people eat less processed food, more fresh fruit and vegetables and using supplements to promote optimal health.

The same is true for dogs. Yes, IBS, allergies, cancers and food intolerances are on the increase in the canine population, too, but nutritional answers to combat these problems are, at best, rather basic. Processed foods still rule. While we humans eat our five pieces of fruit and veg daily, we continue to be brainwashed into feeding processed foods to our dogs. The promise of scientific formulation and convenience lull us into a feeling of 'they know best, so let's just feed the pellets and get on with our lives'.

Does your dog itch too much, get summer skin problems, have frequent loose stools (not diarrhoea, just not easily pick-upable) or recurrent ear infections? If so diet may be the answer. At my holistic veterinary practice I see dogs with these conditions on a daily basis. Introducing them to a raw food diet transforms many. Dogs that have been on steroids for years are able to live drug free lives. Others with histories of years of digestive problems, requiring constant drug treatment, can be symptom free in days or weeks. They never look back.

This whole situation is very simple if you think about it. Dog species have been running around the world's woods and savannahs for millions of years eating a massive variety of fresh game, rotten carcasses, fruit in season, herbivore faeces, grasses and herbs. In the last 20,000 years they've become associated with man and in that time have been exposed to increasingly refined and repetitive diets. In the last 90 years the problem has been compounded with the advent of canning and, more recently, with dried foods for dogs.

The simple answer, therefore, is to give the gut the foods that it was originally designed to digest. This chapter will guide you through a simple raw food diet for dogs that can be easily prepared at home. It offers convenience, broad spectrum nutrition and a means of avoiding, once and for all, processed foods. Your dogs will be healthier, look better, smell better and, above all, enjoy their food much more than the processed foods they have been eating previously.

Meat

Dogs should be fed on a variety of raw meat and bones. Just sticking to one meat source will deprive the dog of nutrients. Do not feed pork. If your dog has a skin or bowel problem, do not initially feed beef; try chicken or turkey or rabbit and wait until you're sure that it won't cause hypersensitivity (4-8 weeks), and then introduce other meats gradually.

For every 10kg of body weight, a dog should eat roughly 100-150g of meat a day. This is only a guideline to start: if your dog is gaining weight, reduce the quantity; if it is losing weight, increase it. Raw chicken wings and turkey necks should be counted as meat, but meaty bones should be fed, in addition to meat, at least twice weekly for teeth cleaning and to supply calcium. Minces with ground bone content are an excellent source of calcium, but will not clean teeth. Only bones, turkey necks or chicken wings, can do this. Twice daily feeding is generally best. Using minced meat is useful because it can be mixed with fruit and veg to induce your dog to eat this component of the diet.

Raw chicken wings or turkey necks can also be fed as part of the meat portion two or three times a week and are ideal for small dogs, large dogs and puppies over 5 weeks. Medium sized dogs are better on turkey necks and large bones.

Never give cooked bones. They are prone to splinter and can cause internal problems for your dog. Raw bones are easily chewed and digested, and provide much-needed calcium and minerals. It is very unlikely, but not impossible, that bones will become stuck in the digestive tract. If you do not give bones to clean teeth, however, poor teeth and general anaesthetics for dental work is very likely (80% of dogs on processed food show gum disease by the age of three). Giving raw vegetable stalks (e.g. broccoli, cabbage, cauliflower) or whole raw carrots and other fibrous vegetables helps to keep teeth clean too.

Proportions

For every handful of meat, feed two handfuls of liquidised raw fruit and veg - a bit like 'meat-and-two-veg' that we're all used to hearing. Freshly ground-up nuts (any nuts), ground-up seeds (pumpkin, sunflower etc), herbs (any except Rosemary) should be added to the 'veg' portion. Cooked beans or sprouted beans can replace meat occasionally. Seeds and nuts are a valuable and very nutritious addition to the diet.

Organ Meat

Feed fresh viscera once a week instead of meat (eg) heart, kidney, lung or liver). Remember, wild animals, as a food source come with viscera as well as muscle meat and bones; it's a necessary part of a balanced diet, however distasteful it may appear to us. Vary the organ meat each week.

Fruit and Vegetables

Take any fruit and vegetables, especially green-leaved ones, fruit and salad items and place in the liquidiser. A good plan is to use some root and some leaf veg in every mix. You can use just two or three ingredients at any one liquidising, but make sure you have variety from week to week.

Blend to a rough broth. If necessary, add some water. Pour the liquidised mix onto the minced meat until you have a meat-to-veg ratio of 1:2 by volume. If your dog is ill or old, you should take a few days to slowly and gradually switch to the new regimen. If they don't like all the veg initially, then start with much more meat for the first week, then wean down, and wean up the veg/fruit mix until you have 30-40% meat, 60-70% veg/fruit mix.

Other Foods:

Treats can include baked liver cubes, small amounts of freeze-dried meats, fruit and veg portions or dried fruit (not raisins). Do not give processed food treats.

Do not feed

Cereals or rice, mixer biscuits or treats. Do not feed raisins, grapes, garlic or onions to dogs as these elements can be toxic.

Do feed

Buckwheat, Amaranth and Quinoa, they are good fillers as they are not cereals. These foods can take the place of rice to add some bulk for hungry dogs.

How to bend the rules:

1. If you cannot bear to feed raw meat, very quick cooking in olive oil to 'seal' the juices is ok. Meat should be rare and cool when served.

2. Liquidised raw veg will last for about forty-eight hours in the fridge, so you need only do the blending three times weekly, although it does begin to lose its goodness pretty soon after liquidising. Rice is fine in small amounts if you're dog is not sensitive to it, but pasta is not good as it is made from wheat.

3. An oven-baked mixer biscuit can be used to fill out the diet once or twice weekly if your dog is not cereal intolerant. Feed one-third meat, one-third veg and one-third high-quality biscuit. Do not use any cereals if you are trying to avoid allergy due to grains.

4 If you really can't bring yourself to feed raw bones or chicken wings, chews should be given to clean the teeth if no bones are fed. Be aware though, that some dogs will be allergic to the rawhide or the pig's ear chews.

Scares

Certain authorities are concerned about feeding dogs raw meat. They claim that such a diet can lead to the dogs becoming infected with bacteria, some that can be passed on to people. In my experience, dogs are naturally able to cope well with the low level of contamination that is present in all fresh uncooked meat. If you have any concerns, or you have very young, very old, or immuno-deficient people in your household, then you would be best advised to talk with your doctor or other health professional.

Supplements

Feeding a raw food diet to your dog, as described here, is the best way to feed, but to ensure they are getting a complete mineral intake, I advise offering a good quality mineral and vitamin supplement. Spirulina can be useful, too. Omega 3 fatty acids such as fish oils or flax seed oils are very healthy. They help with the coat, with any inflammatory condition your dog may have and they promote good organ function. Dogs with arthritis or itching skin, for example, can benefit greatly.

Pups

Puppies need more protein, energy and micronutrients than mature dogs. There are a few modifications to the adult diet that need to be made to meet their greater demands.

Growing pups need more protein than adults. Increase the proportion of meat and chicken wings and turkey necks in the diet to about 50% rather than the 30-40% needed for adults.

Feed pups 3 times daily until they are skeletally mature. That is:

For a Yorkie - about 10-12 months old
For a Springer - about 12-14 months old
For a Labrador - about 14-16 months old
For a Giant breed - over 16 months old.

At maturity, you can gradually reduce the protein level to the adult quantities. Remember, no onions, potatoes or grapes/raisins. You can introduce chicken wings and turkey necks from about six weeks of age.
Pups should be given chicken wings/turkey necks (or bones as they get older) daily.
Avoid beef or tripe products for the first six months. If your pup gets loose on any one meat, just avoid that meat. Organ meat weekly is essential - heart, liver or kidney is very good. If in doubt consult your veterinary surgeon or a veterinary surgeon with knowledge of raw food feeding.

Older Dogs

Feeding older dogs is easier. Use the diet as for the adult dog, but just reduce the protein to about 30% of the total food eaten each day. Increase the fruit and veg component to make up the gap. Otherwise it's exactly the same. Continue with bones and chicken wings, even though their teeth may be absent or worn.

The trouble with changing to the older dog diet is knowing exactly when to do it. This is 'a piece of string' question, I'm afraid. So the guidelines are to use their general vitality - mobility, joie de vie, how keen they are to be involved in the business around the house. As these things reduce, so reduce the protein content of the diet.

Feline nutrition

Cats are not just small dogs - I was taught this at college and it holds true now just as it did then. They are obligate carnivores, for a start. That is, they require a diet very high in protein, unlike dogs. They can only eat fresh meat, unlike the scavenging behaviour of the dog, old and new. From an early age they develop a selective palate, learning early on what is acceptable as 'food' and what is not. Their noses are highly tuned to sniff out anything that is not placed on the menu as a kitten and young cat.

Being so fussy is a protective behaviour. In the wild, if they just ate any old meat like dogs, regardless of its state of decomposition, they would become sick very quickly. They do not have the gastrointestinal defences of dogs and are much more liable to gut infections and toxins.

Taurine, an amino acid found in fresh raw meat, is an essential component of the feline diet. During the 70's and 80's cats were found to be dying of cardiac problems and showing retinal degeneration. Low available Taurine in the processed foods was found to be the culprit. Dogs can synthesise this amino acid, but cats need a steady supply to maintain good health. This is a good example of how cats have evolved a narrow food base orientated around live prey.

A cat will eat its prey whole (except the gall bladder, that is the squidgy green-red thing that the cat leaves for you in the morning if it has been eating a rabbit in the kitchen as you slept soundly upstairs). Wild cats will eat the entire carcass - whole rabbits included. In this way they gain complete nutrition; the prey contains not only all the protein building blocks in muscle and connective tissue, but also fatty acids that are absorbed from fat deposits, nerves and central nervous system tissue.

Where do cats get their carbohydrates from? The gut contents of their herbivore prey. Their rabbit/bird/mouse dinner is full of partially digested grass, cereal or seed and vegetable matter all ready to give the cat the vitamins, fibre, beneficial bacteria and minerals unavailable to it from pure meat sources.

Nature provides the complete meal, ready packaged and keeping fresh out in the neighbouring fields or nearby mouse nest - all ready for a nutritious snack containing all the vitamins and minerals the cat needs, in exactly the right proportions. We need to mimic this food source if we are to breed, raise and maintain healthy domestic cats.

The Holistic Raw Food Diet for Cats

Cats, in my opinion, should eat a raw diet; raw meat, pureed raw fruit and veg and raw chicken wings (for calcium and to clean teeth). It is simple to feed and, logically, it is what cats were, and still are, designed to eat. Here's how it works:

Meat

Cats should be fed on a variety of raw meat and chicken wings. Just sticking to one meat source is no good - you don't get all your nutrients. Poor quality cuts with gristle, bone and a bit of fat are better than pure meat. The best products are those minces that contain minute bone particles. Minces are great because you can mix things with them such as the veg/fruit ration or supplements. They will not have a cleaning effect on the teeth though, so chicken wings and turkey necks are a must. Chicken, turkey, rabbit, lamb, game and beef can all be fed. Feeding in big chunks is better to exercise the jaw and clean the teeth. Do not feed pork.

For every 90-95g of meat, feed 5-10g of pureed raw veg, i.e approximately 95% meat diet with the rest made up of fruit and veg and other non-meat nutrients. Most cats will avoid veg at all costs (although I do know a few who like melon!). By pureeing the food you can smear it on the raw meat or mix with mince which will usually be eaten with gusto. By giving such a small amounts of fruit and veg it is easily hidden. If fruit and veg is impossible for your cat, then seek out good fruit and vegetable based supplements to ensure they get a full spectrum of nutrients. Onions and garlic are toxic to cats - do not feed them.
Quantities - Feed similar quantities as for wet food or twice the volume of dried food previously fed.

Feed raw chicken wings/turkey necks once or twice weekly, minimum. These are highly nutritious and clean teeth very effectively. Cartilage contained helps with joint health, so should be fed from a young age to help with arthritic conditions when older. RAW chicken wings are easily chewed and digested. It is very unlikely, but not impossible, they will get stuck in the gut. If you do NOT give bones to clean teeth, however, a general anaesthetic for dental work is very likely.

Finely ground bone is contained in many chicken, turkey, lamb or rabbit minces. Do check with your supplier as in this way, pet minces are actually superior to human minces bought from a supermarket. Bones give calcium which is essential to bone and general metabolic health.

Feed fresh, non-frozen viscera (kidney, heart, lung or liver) once a week instead of meat. Remember, wild animals come with viscera (organs) alongside the meat. It is a necessary part (however distasteful) of a balanced diet. Vary the organ meat weekly, but make sure heart is often on the menu. Cats, as we have learned, cannot live without Taurine and fresh heart is high in Taurine. Frozen meat has little or no Taurine as the freezing process denatures it, rendering it useless to the cat.

Scares
Certain authorities are concerned with feeding cats raw food. They claim that this can lead to the infection of cats with pathogens that can pass on to people. I believe that cats are able to cope with a certain low level of contamination in their food. I believe they can eat such food and not be more of a threat to human health than a cat fed on a commercial diet. Indeed, if a

cat is fed regularly on a raw food diet, I believe they will be healthier and better able to cope with bugs transmissible to people. If you have any concerns, have very young or very old or immunodeficient people in your household, then your best advice would be to talk with your vet or other health professional.

Fruit and Vegetables

Cats will eat fruit, vegetables, seeds and nuts in the wild in the gut contents of their prey. Vegetables that can be fed to cats include carrots, broccoli, cauliflower, cabbage, swede and any salad items. Fruit can include banana, kiwi fruit, apples, pears, peaches or really anything you can think of. Nuts and seeds should be added to the mix. Nuts could be anything - almonds, walnuts, cashews or hazel nuts, for example are excellent. Seeds include pumpkin or sunflower etc.

Pureeing food

Take the veg, especially green leaved ones, fruit and salad items and place in the liquidiser. You can use just two or three ingredients at any one liquidising, but make sure you have variety from week to week. Add some water to give a liquid texture, if necessary. Blend to a puree and use poured on the meat in a 9 to 1 ratio, meat to veg. You can feed this 2-3 times daily. Do not feed cereals. Do not feed onions and garlic as they are toxic to cats.

Other Foods

Freeze-dried meat or prawns are the only nutritionally acceptable 'treat' for cats. 'Cat milk' is a definite no-no. Your cat was weaned at the age of about six weeks or so, please do not give milk or cat milk.

How to bend the rules above:

1. If you cannot bear to feed raw meat, light cooking in olive oil to 'seal' the juices is ok. Feed as raw as possible.

2. Pureed raw veg will last for 48 hours in the fridge, so you can do the blending only 3x weekly, but remember it loses its goodness pretty quickly after liquidising. Alternatively puree the mix and put into an ice cube tray and freeze - then you can take out small quantities as you need them.

What to do if your cat will not eat raw food

Don't panic, you are not the first owner to have a stubborn cat. But now, at least you know why they are so fussy. They've become fixed on certain types of food, commonly certain brands of dried foods, and now consider anything else to be poison.

With patience, we can usually get round the problem. Firstly, go back to the diet that they are happy on, however unhappy you may be feeding it. Cats are able to starve themselves to death, so don't get into a confrontation situation with them - they will win. Gradually introduce the raw food diet and reduce the old diet. It can take months, but be persistent and crafty in sneaking in the new diet.

Feeding Kittens and Older animals

This is easier than dogs as, essentially, we feed the same diet throughout their lives. Kittens can be offered chicken wings from six to eight weeks and can be offered raw food from before weaning. Feed as for adults, but make sure they have plenty of access to bony material including chicken wings and turkey necks.

Older cats can be fed a slightly lower proportion of meat. Reduce the proportion to about 80% meat, filling the gap with fruit and veg, as for the adult cat.

Equine nutrition

With dogs and cats, we have seen how feeding a diet formulated to suit the evolutionary needs of the animal is logical, healthful and simple. I would like to extend the same principles to horses and ponies.

The majority of horses in the UK are leisure animals in light or medium work such as light hacking, showing, low level dressage or weekend work. They are not expending much more energy than would a horse in the wild. So, it's appropriate to compare the nutrition in the two groups. Of course there are differences in the environment of these two groups, but we can accommodate these in our nutritional decisions.

Polo ponies, eventers and racehorses have an unnaturally high energy requirement. It is beyond the scope of this brief chapter to give details of every horse in every eventuality, so I am concentrating here on the majority of horses, not the elite few.

This large group of leisure horses in the UK are generally poorly fed, even with the best of intentions. Horses and ponies in light or medium work are poorly fed for a number of reasons; access to forage can be limited in stabled animals, energy requirements are overestimated and the weight of the animal is not known for accurate ration measurement. Most horses in this group are over fed, but have poor nutrition.

I'd like to introduce you to a new concept - feeding this group of horses is easy! We will look at the basic ration and then a step by step guide to safely increasing the calorie intake in those animals that tell us they need a little more to do their work. Easy.

Basic Ration

In the wild horses eat long fibre (grass and herbs and weeds) for about 16 hours a day. Domestication by man has not changed this behaviour. If horses and ponies are not chewing for two thirds of the day and night, they are predisposed to vices (wind sucking, box walking or cribbing), especially if their parents had vices. Colic, gastric ulceration and other stress disease are more likely if this simple requirement is not met. So the basic ration must be grass and hay 16 hours a day.

The first thing to do when working out how much to feed your horse is to weigh them. The best weigh tapes are those that take in the girth at the wither and the length of the horse. If they just use the girth, then the margin for error is increased.

Horses should consume between 2 and 2.5 % of their body weight. Warmbloods and ponies should be more at the 2% than the higher end of this range, ponies at the 2.5% end.

So a 300kg pony should be taking in about 6kg (2% body weight) of feed a day (If they're out at grass this is the kind of quantity they would be eating). A relatively light 16hh Thoroughbred type of 500 kg would be on more like 12.5kg (2.5% body weight). For light and medium work, both horses may get by with just forage and feed balancer. If this was not sufficient to maintain weight in the given work and environmental conditions, then the concentrate ration would become 10 then 20 or 30% of this weight. Concentrates should never exceed 30% of the entire ration. It's unlikely that we'd get up to these levels with a leisure animal. If we did, then spread the hard feed ration through the day in two or three meals.

Long Fibre

Grazing

As we're saving you a fortune on buying four different types of supplement and two types of hard feed, I implore you to spend the saving on the best (organic/unsprayed if you can) meadow hay you can find. For good doing animals, get a later cut hay to reduce protein and carbohydrate, for the average horse, earlier cut will help us to keep weight on. Early cut hay should pass the scrunch test - grab a handful and squeeze. If it's spiky, then it's a bit late cut; a bit fibrous, and an earlier cut would be better.

Greenness is not a good indicator of nutritional value, but softness is. Hay should be clean, dust free and without a mouldy smell. It should be soaked for only five or ten minutes before feeding to reduce leaching of water soluble nutrients. Always feed from the ground where possible - this is where horses have been grazing for millions of years. Why change it now for our convenience?

Haylage is a good alternative to hay, but care must be taken to use the bale quickly to prevent spoiling and toxic bacterial and mould contamination once the seal is broken. Consume, ideally within 24 - 36 hours. Good for dust/mould allergic horses.

Medieval pasture, so I'm told, used to contain over 27 varieties of grass, flower and herb. Modern leys are lucky if they top seven. A great diversity of plant life provides diversity of nutrition because a variety of plants have a variety of nutritional value. But it also uses the soil more thoroughly and effectively. Dandelions, for example have deep tap roots that can pull minerals up from deep soil strata. The Timothies and the Rye grasses of this world can literally only scrape the surface.

Modern farming, using nitrogen fertilisers, produce very green and lush grass, but if this has been harvested year after year when only nitrogen and potash has been applied, then it's just mathematics to determine that it will be available-mineral poor. Feed balancers are the answer.

Feed Balancers

Feed balancers are combination products that allow the basic 16 hour-a-day long-fibre feral horse diet accommodate to modern life. Firstly, they contain minerals and vitamins to balance and complement those found in a basic ration. This makes up for the fact we keep our horses in limited acreage, not the prairies and savannahs they evolved in where broad nutrition was available from the ground.

Pro-biotics are beneficial bacteria that help to re-equilibrate the gut after stress or antibiotic treatment. Having lots of good bugs in the gut is a good idea as it gives less room for the bad bugs to get a toe-hold.

Pre-biotics are starchy substances (such as manno-oligosaccharide) that feed the resident gut bacteria to enhance their cellulose digestion and vitamin production activity, for example.

Saccharomyces cerevisiae (bakers/brewer's yeast) is a yeast that the gut bacteria really relish. It promotes regulation of acidity, vitamin production and the overall running of the bugs in the gut, so it's as well to keep them happy.

When choosing a feed balancer I go for one which, as well as being high in nutrients, is cereal free, dairy free and non-GM if possible. To this, I would add succulents such as apple, carrot or swede etc. to improve palatability. Often horses will eat the balancer on its own or will get to like the taste quite quickly without the treats added. If they really don't like it, then apple or orange juice can work wonders!

The Energy Ladder

So there we have it - how to feed most of the light and medium working horses with just two products; long fibre and a feed balancer. This is fantastic in all but older animals and those animals that tend to worry or work off any weight they put on. For them, we have a graded list of additions to the simple duo above. We do this to use the most calorific and least potentially damaging energy foods first, saving the cereals until we have no choice but to use them to maintain weight and provide energy for work. Changes to the diet should be made gradually. It takes the gut 10 days to alter itself to any new feedstuff, so a 10 day introduction period for any change should always be aimed for. If you change 10% of the diet each day for this period, it will reduce the chance of colics, laminitis and tying-up problems.

The list should be read from top to bottom. Start your horse or pony on the top of the list and go down the list, adding each to the diet until you have sufficient energy going in to maintain weight. If they are putting on weight or are over weight, you can use the list backwards to gradually withdraw energy foods, starting with the worst and finishing with the least bad. Remember - concentrates should be fed little and often.

With all concentrated feeds, start with a small amount and assess the effect on condition and sparkle in work after one to two weeks.

Forage - increase energy from forage by feeding more of what you're already feeding or then move to a higher energy forage e.g. Alfalfa or a dried grass product or grass nuts/cubes.

Oil - add soya, corn or olive oil (or alternating them is even better) to the feed balancer to provide non fermentable calories. Oil is absorbed in the small intestine, so does not negatively affect the fermentation in the hind gut. Feed up to 2-3 cups a day for a horse, half this for a pony. This is all that most ponies need to maintain weight. The side effect is a great looking coat! If you feed too much, you'll just see greasy or slightly sloppy droppings. If you see this, reduce the oil a bit until this disappears. Top Spec produce a Super Conditioning Flake that is high in oil. It can eliminate the necessity of adding liquid oil to concentrates. It is very palatable and can be used for horses that don't like a greasy meal.

Non-molassed Beet Pulp - again, this is non cereal calories, but does reach the hind gut where it is digested to provide fuel energy.

Whole Oats - yes, they are cereals, but if fed as in small quantities (1-2 cups with each meal), and soaked over-night, then they really are not heating. Bruised oats are also a good form of oats.

Cereal free Cool mix - based on grasses or other long fibre and added oils. Be careful here because these products can have added minerals and vitamins and this can then double up on the adequate supply of these nutrients by the feed balancer.

Straights - e.g micronised barley can be fed in addition to oats, but is usually fed in place of these. Some horses will do better and be less heated by using barley rather than oats. My preference is usually to go for oats first.

Cereal Mix - e.g endurance or racing nuts/cubes or pencils. These are reserved for those horses that are just not getting by and delivering good work and maintaining weight when all the other elements of the list have been tried.

Summer and Winter Feeding

In the wild, horses would get fatter in the summer and thinner in the winter. I feel this is a good cycle to model your horse on. Over the summer they may well gain condition because of the abundance of grass, but the trick is to let them gradually lose this during the winter. In this way fat soluble toxins stored in the fat deposits can be shed and then replenished annually. We don't want them to run off to skeletons by Christmas; the guidelines are to aim for fat and fit at the end of the summer and trim and fit at the end of winter. I don't think that maintaining a constant weight is healthy for any mammal. That includes humans!

contents

Algae: Spirulina	66-68
Aloe Vera	61
Angelica root	87
Animal Aromatics - is it safe?	12
Animal Aromatics is not aromatherapy	10
Arnica flowers	78
Aromatic Waters	69
Base oils frequency chart	38
Base oils	61-63
Base oils: how to decide which to use	38
Basil, French	88
Bay Laurel	89
Beeswax	63-64
Behaviour changes to animals	22
Bergamot	90-91
Beta carotenes	75
Birch yellow	148
Caged animals	42
Canine: ear infections	180
Canine: gum disease / toothpaste	183
Canine: joint problems	181-182
Canine: skin Problems	182-183
Canine : taking large amounts of fatty oils	178-179
Canine: travelling	183
Canine: tumours / warts / lumps	183
Canine: what to do if all macerated are liked	178
Canine: wounds	180
Canine – case studies	184-191
Canine: remedies frequently selected	177
Carrot macerated	79
Carrot seed essential oil: a dog bitten by a rattlesnake	9
Carrot seed, wild	92-93
Cat rescue centre	200-205
Cat: stress related cystitis	49
Catnip flowers	70
Cats: arthritis	195
Cats: cystitis	195
Cats: grooming	194
Cats: how to offer their remedies	193
Cats: indoor	193
Cats: thyroid problems	194

Cats: wounds	194
Chalk	71
Chamomile, German	94-95
Chamomile, Roman	96-97
Chart: Oils for common disorders	59-60
Chickweed	79
Clary Sage	98
Clay	64-65
Clay: essential oils added	39
Colic : Horse	36
Colic	163
Comfrey	80
Convulsions / fits	154
Devil's claw	72
Dilutions	36-40
Dog: fear of men	49
Dog: prostate problem	48
Dogs: Labrador with faded pigmentation	14
Dying	157
Equine – case studies	168-176
Equine: boxing: Problems	167
Equine: fly repellent	165
Equine: invigorating rub	167
Equine: Remedies frequently selected	159
Equine: rub down	167
Equine: splints	166
Equine: travel rub	167
Equine: travelling	166
Equine: wounds	160
Equine: sun screen	166
Essential fatty acids (EFAs)	76
Essential oil adulteration	27
Essential oil care	28
Eucalyptus	99-100
Extraction	24-26
Feline – case studies	196-199
Feline: remedies frequently selected	192
Fennel common / bitter	101
Fennel sweet	101
Flax or linseed oil	83
Fleas / mites / midges	156
Flouve	102
Frankincense	103
Frequency: of selected macerated oils	77
Frequency: of offering remedies	42
Garlic	104-106
Gels: How to prepare	38-39
Geranium	107
Healing Crisis - behavioural - horse	35
Heart / mind / behavioural problems	54
Hemp seed oil	84
Hoof moisturiser	165

Hoof	52	Neem oil	85
Horse selecting remedies – example	47-48	Nutmeg	120
Immortelle	108	Observation	33-34
Immune problems and allergies	57	Olfaction	20
Insect bites	155	Oral administration	23
Jasmine Absolute	109	Orange Blossom / Neroli	121
Joint problems	161	Peppermint	122-123
Juniper Berry	110-111	Photosensitisation	14
Kidney and bladder	53	Pink Lotus	124
Laminitis	162	Plants and mammals	10
Large intestine	51	Plants that cause a reaction can treat that same reaction	13
Lavender	112-113	Primary and secondary metabolites	11
Lemon	114	Quality: The importance of quality	26
Lemongrass	115	Rain scald	164
Licorice root (powder)	73	Remedies - offering	31-32
Lime	116	Remedies – selecting	30
Linden blossom macerate	80	Ringworm	155
Linden blossom absolute	117	Rose	125-127
Liver and gall bladder	55	Rosehips-dried fruit, and CO_2	73-74
Lungs	50	Rosemary	128
Macerated oils	76	'Safe'	16
Mange	156	Safety notes	29
Marigold	81	Sandalwood	129-130
Marjoram Sweet	118	Sea Buckthorn	131-132
Mud fever	164	Seaweed	133-136
Mugwort, Great	119		

Secondary compounds in the feed?	17
Skin	51
Spearmint	137
Spikenard	138
Spleen and stomach	56
St John's wort	81-82
Summary: offering remedies	86
Summary: remedies and dilutions	43-45
Summary: responses	46
Sweet itch	163
Tea Tree	139-141
Thrush	164
Thyme	142-143
Topical application	41
Topical use of essential oils	22
Toxicity	15
Tumours / sarcoids / warts	162
Valerian	144
Vanilla	145
Vetiver	146
Violet Leaf Absolute	147
Viruses, fungi and bacteria	18-19
Vomeronasal organ	21
Water	65
Water: essential oils added	39
Wheat grass (powder)	74
Wintergreen	148
Wintergreen: a pony selects wintergreen	16
Yarrow	149-150
Ylang Ylang	151

references

Introduction: A step by Step Guide: Organ Systems of the body: Base Materials

[1] Engel, C (2002) Wild Health. Weidenfeld & Nicolson: London

[2] Ker Than www.livescience.com/blogs/author/kerthan LiveScience Staff Writerposted: 10 July 2006

[3] McTaggart, L (2001) The Field. The Quest of the Secret Force of the Universe. HarperCollins Publishers: London

[4] Martens, A et al. (2000) In vitro and in vivo evaluation of hypericin for photodynamic therapy of equine sarcoids. The Veterinary Journal 159(1):77-84

[5] Ingraham, T (2006) A comparative investigation into the antibacterial effects of a variety of essential oils and antibiotics on three strains of Escherichia coli bacteria. Clifton College science department.

[6] Author names. (1992) Article title. The Journal of Cancer Research and Clinical Oncology page numbers

[7] Yang, S (2005) Got kelp? New UC Berkeley research finds that seaweed can reduce level of hormone related to breast cancer risk. http://sph.berkeley.edu/research/highlights/05feb02.htm

[8] Watson, L (2001) Jacobson's organ and the Remarkable Nature of Smell. A Plume Book: Published by the Penguin Books Ltd. London

[9] Jager et al. (1996) Pharmokinetic studies of the fragrance compound 1,8-cineole in humans during inhalation. Chemical Senses 21 (4): 477-479

[10] Gwaltney-Brant et al. (2001) Differing opinions of raw food diet research…Renal failure associated with ingestion of grapes or raisins in dogs. Journal of the American Veterinary Medical Association. 218 (10): 1553-1556

[11] Wells, D (2006) Aloe Vera Gel. Animal Aromatics course paper

[12] Ryrie, C. (1998) The Healing Energies of Water. Gaia Books: London

[13] VeganHealth.org

http://www.veganhealth.org/articles/iodine

Macerates

[1] Kozlenko, R, Henson, R H (1998) Latest scientific research on spirulina: Effects on the Aids Virus, Cancer and the Immune System. www.spirulina.com/SPLNews96.html

[2] Loseva, L P, Dardynskaya, I V(1993) Spirulina - natural sorbent of radionucleides. Research Institute of Radiation Medicine, Minsk, Belarus. 6th International Congress of Applied Algology, Czech Republic.

[3] Engel, C (2002) Wild Health. Weidenfeld & Nicolson: London

[4] The Merck Manuals Online Medical Library. Calcium: www.merck.com/mmhe/sec12/ch155/ch155b.html?qt=calcium&alt=sh#sec12-ch155-ch155b-231 accessed 01/08/06

[5] Green, D (2004) Devil's claw. Animal Aromatics course paper

[6] Tilford, G L (1997) Edible and Medicinal Plants of the West. Cited in: Botany in a Day (2000) Thomas J. Elpel's Herbal Field Guide to Plant Families. 4th edition. Hops Press: Montana, USA

[7] Shiki Y et al (1992) Effect of glycyrrhizin on lysis of hepatocyte membranes induced by anti-liver cell membrane antibody. J Gastroenterol Hepatol. 7(1):12-6

[8] Hoffman, D L. Liquorice. http://www.healthy.net/scr/article.asp?ID=1408 accessed 01/08/06

[9] Wildcrafted Herbal Products. Medicinal Herb; Licorice (Glycyrrhiza glabra) www.wildcrafted.com.au/Botanicals/Licorice.html. Accessed: 29/07/06

[10] Davis, S (2004) Wheat grass. Animal Aromatics course paper

[11] Arnica montana L. Plants for a future database report. http://www.pfaf.org/database/plants.php?Arnica+montana. Accessed 01/08/06

[12] Self, H P (1996) Modern Horse Herbal. Kenilworth Press: Buckingham

[13] Degar, S et al (1992) Inactivation of the human immunodeficiency virus by hypericin: evidence for photochemical alterations of p24 and a block in uncoating. AIDS Res Hum Retroviruses 8 (11): 1929-1936

[14] Adlercreutz, H (2002) Phyto-oestrogens and cancer. Lancet Oncology 3 (6): 364-373

[15] Centre for Indian Knowledge systems. Preparation of neem biopesticides at farm level. http://tcdc.undp.org/sie/experiences/vol4/Neem%20biopesticides.pdf. Accessed: 28/07/06

[16] Biswas, K et al (2002) Biological activities and medicinal properties of neem (Azadirachta indica). Current Science 82(11):1336-1345

Essential oil profiles References/ Bibliography

[1] Hao, Y Y, Bracket, R E, Doyle, M P (1998) Efficacy of plant extracts in inhibiting Aeromonas hydrophila and Listeria monocytogenes in refrigerated, cooked poultry. Food Microbiology 15 (4): 367-378

[2] Aruna K, Sivaramakrishnan, V M (1996) Anticarcinogenic effects of the essential oils from cumin, poppy and basil. Phytotherapy Research 10 (7): 577-580

[3] Occhiuto F, Circosta C (1996) Antianginal and antiarrhythmic effects of bergamottine, a furocoumarin isolated from bergamot oil. Phytotherapy Research 10 (6): 491-496

[4]Tisserand R, Balacs, T (1995) Essential Oil Safety. A Guide for Health Care Professionals. Churchill Livingstone: Edinburgh

[5] Martens, A et al. (2000) Researched In Vitro and In Vivo Evaluation of Hypericin for Photodynamic Therapy of Equine Sarcoids. The Veterinary Journal 159 (1):77-84

[6] Elegbede, J A et al. (1986) Regression of rat mammary tumors following dietary d-limonene. J. Natl. Cancer Inst. 76, 323-325.

[7] Chen I S et al. (1996) Coumarins and antiplatelet aggregation constituents from Formosan Peucedanum japonicum. Phytochemistry 41(2): 525-530

[8] Valnet, J (1980) The Practice of Aromatherapy. C W Daniel Company Ltd: Saffron Walden

[9] Yamada K et al. (1996) Effect of inhalation of chamomile oil vapour on plasma ACTH level in ovariectomized rat under restriction stress. Biological & Pharmaceutical Bulletin 19 (9): 1244-1246

[10] Battaglia, S (1995) The Complete Guide to Aromatherapy. (First edition) Perfect Potion: Virginia QLD.

[11] Schnaubelt, K (1998) Advanced Aromatherapy. The Science of Essential Oil Therapy. Healing Arts Press: Vermont

[12] Tisserand R (1977) The Art of Aromatherapy. C W Daniel Company Ltd: Saffron Walden

[13] Ih-Sheng C et al (1996) Coumarins and anti-platelet aggregation constituents from Formosan Peucedanum japonicum. Phytochemistry 41:525-530

[14] Yardley, A (2004) A preliminary study investigating the effect of the application of some essential oils on the in vitro proliferation of Dermatophilus congolensis. International Journal of Aromatherapy 14 (3): 129-135

[15] Asham M, et al. (1996) Garlic extract and allicin: broad spectrum agents effective against multiple drug resistant strains of Shigella dysenteriae type 1 and Shigella flexneri, enterotoxigenic Escherichia coli and Vibrio cholerae. Phytotherapy Research 10 (4): 329-331

[16] Burger R A et al. (1993) Enhancement of in vitro immune function by Allium sativum L. (garlic) fractions. International Journal of Pharmacognosy.

[17] Ashan, M, Islam, S N (1996) Garlic: a broad-spectrum antibacterial agent effective against common pathogenic bacteria. Fitotherapia 67 (4) 374-376

[20] Black's Veterinary Dictionary (1928) Edited by Miller WC. The Waverley Book Company: London

[21] Stassi V (1996) The antimicrobial activity of the essential oil of four Juniperus species growing wild in Greece. Flavour and Fragrance Journal 11:71-74

[22] Leung, AY, Foster, S (1996) Encyclopedia of Common Natural Ingredients Used in Food, Drugs and Cosmetics. Second edition. John Wiley & Sons Inc: New York

[23] Guba, R (1999) Toxicity Myths…The actual risks of Essential Oil use. Part II. Aromatherapy Today 12: 16-21

[24] Schilcher, H, Leuschner, F (1997) Studies of potential nephrotoxic effects of essential juniper oil. Arzneimittelforschung 47 (7): 855

[25] Tisserand, R (1977) The Art of Aromatherapy. C W Daniel Company Ltd: Saffron Walden

[26] Kawakami, M, Aoki, S, Ohkubo, T (1999) A study of fragrance on working environment characteristics in VDT work activities. International Journal of Production Economics 60-61: 575-581

[28] Lorenzetti, B B et al. (1991) Myrcene mimics the peripheral analgesic activity of lemongrass tea. Journal of Ethnopharmacology 34 (1): 43-48

[29] Tisserand, R, Balacs, T (1995) Essential Oil Safety. A Guide for Health Care Professionals. Churchill Livingstone: Edinburgh

[30] Bennett, A et al.(1988) The biological activity of eugenol, a major constituent of nutmeg (Myristica fragrans): studies on prostaglandins, the intestine and other tissues. Phytotherapy Research 2 (3): 124-130

[31] Rees W D, Evans B K, Rhodes J (1979)Treating irritable bowel syndrome with peppermint oil. British Medical Journal 2 (6194): 835-836

[32] Gobel H et al. (1995) Essential plant oils and headache mechanisms. Phytomedicine 2 (2): 93-102

[33] Mojay, G (1996) Aromatherapy for Healing the Spirit. Gaia Books Ltd: London

[34] Stahl, W et al. (2000) Carotenoids and carotenoids plus vitamin E protect against ultraviolet light-induced erythema in humans. Am J Clin Nutr. 71:795-798.

[35] Nishino, H et al (2002) Carotenoids in Cancer Chemoprevention. Cancer and Metastasis Reviews. 12(3-4): 257-264

[36] Ellouali M et al (1993) Antitumor activity of low molecular weight fucans extracted from brown seaweed Ascophyllum nodosu. Anticancer Research 16 (6A): 2011-2019

[37] UK Food Guide. A guide to additives in and on our food. E400 Alginic Acid. http://www.ukfoodguide.net/e400.htm accessed: 01/08/06

[39] Olsen, C B (1998) Australian Tea Tree Oil. Kali Press: Pagosa Springs, CO.

[40] Villar, D et al. (1994) Toxicity of melaleuca oil and related essential oils applied topically on dogs and cats. Vet Human Toxicol 36 (2): 139-142

[41] Durant, S, Karran, P (2003) Vanillins - a novel family of DNA-PK inhibitors. Nucleic Acids Research 31 (19): 5501-5512

[42] Gattefosse, R-M, Tisserand, R (ed) (1993) Gattefosse's Aromatherapy. C W Daniel Company Ltd Saffron: Walden

[43] Betts, T (2003) Semiochemistry workshop. Imperial College, London.

[44] Herb Research Foundation. Herbworld News Online. Research reviews: http://www.herbs.org/current/sjwvsbestsellers.htm Accessed: 01/08/06